Contents

16 The handicapped adolescent   209

PART III   Treatment and management of the disturbed
                 adolescent   233
17 The first interview and principles of treatment   235
18 Physical methods of treatment in adolescent psychiatry   241
19 Psychological   methods   of   treatment   in   adolescent
       psychiatry   264
20 Social intervention and residential provision in adolescence   282
21 The adolescent in-patient   295
22 Conclusion   302

        Envoi   304

        Index   305

GRO

a stud   stress

Edna M. Irwin

Consultant Psychiatrist
Hollymoor Hospital,
Birmingham

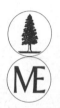

MACDONALD AND EVANS

MACDONALD & EVANS LTD.
Estover, Plymouth PL6 7PZ

First published 1977

© Edna M. Irwin 1977

ISBN 0 7121 0724 X

Text set in 11/12 pt Photon Times, printed by photolithography,
and bound in Great Britain at The Pitman Press, Bath

Editor's Foreword

Working with adolescents is never easy, as any school teacher will confirm. Working with psychiatrically-disturbed adolescents is a highly complex and demanding task, which requires a certain type of dedication which relatively few people possess. This is true of all the personnel concerned, whether they be from psychiatric, social work, nursing or other disciplines. People who can work successfully with the disturbed adolescent are, therefore, a highly selected group and the group is quite a small one. However, although their numbers are small, their work is very important. This is a fairly new field and it is one about which people, either professional or lay, know very little. Therefore, it seems right to illumine this area for the non-specialist and this is what Dr. Irwin has set out to do in this book, in my opinion, highly successfully.

Adolescents have always been with us, but there is still a tendency to regard them as overgrown children or under-developed adults. Lip-service is paid to the concept that they have problems specific to themselves, but when these problems become acute, frequently there are no facilities available to help them and attempts are made to squeeze the adolescent into some inappropriate therapeutic mould. Fortunately, this situation is beginning to change and there is increasing interest and concern for their welfare.

I have said that work with them is important and I would reiterate this. Adolescence is a kind of psychiatric crossroad, at which a number of serious disorders may appear and the earlier they can be recognised and treated the better; on the other hand, it is also a time at which the effects of unduly harmful events occurring in childhood may still be undone and much positive benefit brought about for the individual's future mental health. So, it can be viewed as a period when, at least potentially, useful interventive and preventive work may be carried out.

As Dr. Irwin points out, despite the many problems of being a teenager, most adolescents are remarkably healthy and it is a small minority who require psychiatric help. But, untended disorders at this age may produce a very prolonged period of ill-health and malfunctioning, with severe repercussions on the family, the school and the various other organisations with which the disturbed individual comes in contact. Society itself may suffer, since not too infrequently, teenage disturbance may overflow into delinquency and other anti-social behaviours. A great deal of crime is committed these days by youngsters, including a sizeable proportion of violent crime. These phenomena will not disappear of their own accord and our habit of trying to ignore them is wearing very thin at present.

Adolescents always seem to create more problems than their numbers justify. This is common knowledge and it applies to psychiatric illness just as much as to anything else. But if you were to judge how important psychiatric disorder of adolescence was from its representation in standard textbooks, you would be forced to conclude that it was quite a minor cause for concern. Or, if you were to consider how little there is in the general literature that is truly informative about adolescence, normal and abnormal, you might decide that perhaps you were mistaken and that teenagers, after all, lived a singularly uneventful life!

We know this is not true. A growing number of professional and voluntary workers are developing a rapidly increasing awareness of, and expertise in, the psychological problems of this particular age group. As one of the small group of adolescent psychiatrists, and as leader of an inter-disciplinary therapeutic team, Dr. Irwin is in an excellent position to provide us with an overview of her subject and she has done this well. Her book was designed especially for those interested in the social work aspects of adolescent mental disorders and I am confident that it will fill an increasingly noticeable gap in the literature for workers in this area. In addition, she has much to say of interest and common sense that will be of value to the involved layman (including the interested parent) at one end, and the nurse, medical practitioner, psychologist and school teacher at the other. I learned a great deal from her book and enjoyed her 'sense and sensibility' approach, as I am quite sure you, the reader, will do.

Alistair Munro
Toronto, 1977

Preface

On opening a hospital unit for emotionally disturbed adolescents, the author was faced with an in-service training programme for a multi-disciplinary staff team. The senior nurses at the unit had State Registration in psychiatric and general nursing, but had no knowledge of child and adolescent development. The occupational therapist was in a similar situation. The teachers had knowledge of child and adolescent development, but were ill-equipped to deal with some of the psychiatric problems with which they were presented. As the unit became established, students from various disciplines rotated through the unit, and it was difficult to provide them with the information that they wished to have within the short space of time that they were attached to the adolescent unit. Information was available, but it was widely scattered in books and journals and, therefore, not easily accessible. The ensuing chapters are the outcome of the author's attempts to minimise the gaps between the various disciplines and provide a basic text for workers in this area.

As with other residential establishments for disturbed youngsters, hospital adolescent units rely heavily on the untrained, mature adult. With time, such staff acquire a sophisticated knowledge about the emotional problems of adolescence, but their introduction to an adolescent unit can be a threatening experience, as they have little idea of what to expect. Whilst no extensive knowledge is required to have some awareness of the nature and treatment of common physical ailments, for example, appendicitis, cancer and diabetes, even well-informed lay people have little knowledge of the different types of psychiatric illness and assume that all mental illness is associated with a sinister prognosis. New staff find themselves at a loss to answer questions posed by a young patient, and staff ignorance contributes to feelings of insecurity amongst both staff and patients. The ensuing chapters are an attempt to reduce this unawareness.

As there is a considerable literature available on child care, social work and education, the author has chosen to confine herself to the more specifically psychiatric aspects of teenage disturbance, so that many areas of concern, such as teenage violence, are not considered. To a large extent, the writer has adhered to the so-called 'medical model' in which a clinical history is used to make a diagnosis; on the basis of this, treatment is prescribed and a prognosis is made. Some repetition between chapters is deliberate, so that if, for example, a teacher is presented with a pupil who is considered to suffer from anorexia nervosa the appropriate chapter may be consulted. To facilitate access to further knowledge, references and a selection of further reading is appended at the end of each chapter.

Since the influences of childhood have a considerable bearing on the subsequent development of the adolescent and the adult, it seemed appropriate to examine briefly pre-adolescent development, but the main body of the text relates to adolescent psychological development and deviation. As this is an introductory text, treatment has been covered only briefly, details of techniques being beyond the scope of this work. An exception has been made in the area of physical methods of treatment in psychiatry, as it was considered that an understanding of techniques and a detailed account of the drugs used in psychiatry, with their side effects, might be of value, particularly to teachers and social workers. Except where specifically indicated, the pronoun 'he' has been used throughout, instead of the more cumbersome 'he/she'.

E.I.
Birmingham, March 1977

PART I
NORMAL DEVELOPMENT

1 Nature and nurture

Personality is defined in the *Shorter Oxford English Dictionary* as 'that assemblage of qualities which makes a person unique'. Mature adult personality arises from a combination of factors derived from nature and nurture.

Nature:
1. Genetic endowment.
2. Physical (biological) factors.

Nurture:
1. Psychological influences contributed from the child's immediate environment, *e.g.* the home, school.
2. The wider socio-cultural environment in which the child grows up.

Let us consider these factors in some detail.

NATURE

The pre-natal stage
Conception of the future individual takes place when the sperm cell of the father penetrates the ovum (egg) within the mother—a

3

process called fertilisation. Over the next nine months, the fertilised
ovum divides, divides again and again, each time doubling in size,
to form the two-cell, four-cell, eight-cell stages, etc. As development
proceeds, the various body tissues, for example, skin, muscle and
cartilage, and the rudimentary organs, including the heart tube, the
kidney tube and the neural (nerve) tube, become recognisable with
a high-powered microscope. As it increases in size and complexity,
the developing organism becomes known, successively, as the embryo and then the foetus. In the human being, for the first forty
weeks of life from conception until birth, development normally
takes place in the uterus (womb) of the mother, and we refer to this
as the pre-natal period of life. (The Chinese acknowledge these forty weeks, so that at birth the Chinese infant is said to be one year
old.) A baby born before forty weeks is premature. It is rare for an
infant to survive if it is born before the twenty-eighth week of intra-
uterine life. Babies weighing less than 2,500 g are light or
premature. Underweight babies may be born at term, when they
are described as 'light for dates', rather than premature. Very low
birth weight may be associated with later physical and emotional
problems.

During the period of intra-uterine existence, the foetus is
nourished from the mother's blood-stream through the placenta
(which becomes the after-birth)—tissue which is attached to the
wall of the uterus. Blood vessels pass through the placenta to the
foetus, forming the umbilical cord. Should the placenta become
detached from the uterine wall there is interference with foetal
nutrition, and there may be insufficient oxygen to maintain life.
Vaginal haemorrhage may be an indication of placental separation.
If the interference with foetal nutrition is serious, the foetus may die
and a still-birth results (before the twenty-eighth week of intra-
uterine life, death of the foetus is termed abortion, or miscarriage).
If the foetus survives the mishap, there may be brain damage.

Sometimes, if the health of the mother is affected, that of the
foetus may be affected also. The tragedies which resulted when
expectant mothers took the drug thalidomide are fairly recent and
well known. Most mothers are aware of the risk of a baby being
born blind, deaf, or having heart disease, should they suffer from
German measles during the early stages of pregnancy. Excessive
irradiation (X-ray examination or treatment) may result in deformity

of the developing embryo. In addition to damage to the foetus mediated through the mother, difficulties may arise during the birth process when, for short periods, the foetus may be deprived of oxygen. If the oxygen-lack is severe there may be damage to the nervous system, particularly to the cells in the brain stem. Seriously affected children may be found to have paralysis of a limb, or limbs, or tremulous movements, conditions included in the term cerebral palsy ('spastic').

Difficulties during labour and delivery may further handicap the new born infant.

Some of the factors which I have been describing, have been examined by Knobloch, Pasamanick and Lilienfeld who have developed *a theory of the continuum of reproductive casualty*. In essence, they suggest that, at conception, a future individual is as nearly 'perfect' as that individual can be, but in the process of development, before, during and after birth, a series of damaging influences may make him rather less perfect than nature had intended at the outset. Advances in medical knowledge have resulted in the survival of many handicapped infants who formerly would have died soon after birth, but perhaps the most amazing feature of all is that, despite the many ways in which development can go wrong before birth, there are relatively few defective humans.

Genetic influences

When the sperm and ovum combine to form the zygote (the fertilised ovum), each contributes to the genetic endowment of the future individual. Virtually every human has forty-six chromosomes, which are located in the nucleus of the human cell as twenty-three pairs, one of each pair being contributed by the father and the other by the mother. One pair of chromosomes is known as the sex chromosomes, and the others are non-sex chromosomes, or autosomes. Chromosomes contain factors known as genes, which carry the attributes which a child inherits from his parents. With the use of the electron microscope, we are learning more about chromosomes and the occasional structural abnormalities which can arise. Each pair of autosomes is of equal length, and this is also true of female sex chromosomes, but in the male, the sex chromosomes are unequal in length. Female sex chromosomes are known as 'X' chromosomes and every normal female has two 'X' chromosomes, so that in reproduction, when contributing to the chromosomal constitution of the next generation, the mother can only donate an 'X' chromosome. The male chromosomes are the large 'X' chromosome and the smaller 'Y' chromosome, the 'X' being obtained from the mother and the 'Y' from the father. In his turn, the male can donate an 'X' chromosome to the next generation, thus siring a daughter, or a 'Y' chromosome, when the progeny will be male, that is it is the father's contribution which determines the sex of the next generation. (Interestingly, husbands have been known to berate their wives when, time after time, a child of the same sex has been born!) It is fascinating to think that every single cell in the human body is either male or female according to the sex of the individual. The vulnerability of the human male has long been recognised; for example, it is known that more male offspring abort spontaneously, and also die in the first year of life; it is widely recognised the female longevity exceeds that of males, although females tend to have poorer health in adult life. (One suggestion has been that this male vulnerability may be related to the inequality of the length of the sex chromosomes in the male.) Until puberty, female development tends to be ahead of that of males and for example, girls learn to speak and read in advance of boys, even when allowance is made for intellectual differences, and of course puberty occurs earlier in girls.

Chromosomal abnormalities occur; these may be numerical or structural and may involve the sex chromosomes or the autosomes. Many chromosomal abnormalities are incompatible with survival and spontaneous abortion occurs. Perhaps the best known chromosomal abnormality is Down's Syndrome (Mongolism), also known as trisomy 21, in which the infant has 47 chromosomes, the additional one being associated with the pair of autosomes designated '21'. Surveys have now been carried out to assess the chromosomal constitution of new-born infants. A study in Edinburgh (Ratcliffe *et al*) of 3,500 new-born male infants, revealed that twenty had an abnormal chromosomal constitution. Eight of these had a sex chromosomal abnormality and in eleven it was an autosomal abnormality.

The genes carried by the chromosomes are composed of the chemical deoxyribonucleic acid (D.N.A.) and thousands of genes are arranged on each chromosome. Over a hundred years ago,

Gregor Mendel, an Austrian monk, was able to formulate a theory regarding the transmission of heredity, as a result of his observations on two strains of peas. Certain attributes were transmitted more frequently to the next generation than others. These Mendel recognised as dominant features and the less frequently transmitted traits as recessive features. From these observations, the comparison of attributes of identical and non-identical twins, with advances in technical skills, and an increase in the knowledge of human biochemistry, we are becoming more aware of the complexity of heredity and are recognising which characteristics are inherited. However, the environment interacts with inherited features. For example, it is recognised that the potential for height is inherited, but if there is dietary insufficiency, an individual cannot attain his full potential. Similarly, the current view is that intelligence is largely inherited, but obviously education, using the term in its widest sense, is required to enable the individual to make full use of his intelligence.

Some diseases are genetically determined, for example certain forms of mental deficiency such as phenylketonuria, which results from an inborn error of metabolism, in which a particular enzyme required in the metabolism of a protein, phenylalanine, found in many substances, is missing. This is a recessive feature, so that approximately one progeny in four will be affected, when both parents are carriers of the abnormal gene. The recognition of genetic or chromosomal abnormalities is important in our understanding of abnormalities, but as yet we cannot tackle the problems directly by physically altering the genetic constitution.

Direct evidence of genetic factors influencing disease is unavailable, and indirect evidence difficult to obtain. As yet, we are unaware of the extent to which genetic factors contribute to personality. A particularly interesting prospective longitudinal study carried out in New York has contributed to our knowledge in this area. Doctors Thomas, Chess, Birch and their co-workers, followed up over one hundred children of professional parents from the earliest months of infancy to early school days by direct observation, diaries kept by parents and interviews with parents. From these sources, a behavioural style (temperament) was described for each child. Nine categories of behavioural reactions were used and children were rated, on scales, as falling at one or other extreme or middle. Analysis of the ratings of the children from these nine categories suggested that there were five groups of traits:

1. The regular, adaptable child, exhibiting mild intensity, approach and positive mood.
2. The irregular, non-adaptable child, who reacted with high intensity, withdrawal, negative mood and high activity.
3. The moderately adaptable child, exhibiting mild intensity, withdrawal and negative mood, low or moderate activity level.
4. The child with a low threshold of response, distractible, with a short attention-span and low persistence.
5. The child with a high threshold of response and non-distractibility.

As the children grew, a proportion presented to the psychiatrist with clinical problems. It was noted that the temperamental pattern which produced the greatest risk of behavioural problems in development was that of the child who was irregular in biological function, having a predominantly negative response to new stimuli, with slow adaptability to change, frequent negative moods and a predominantly intense reaction (Group 2). This child was the difficult baby who made considerable demands on the adaptability of his parents. It is interesting that Chess comments that the parents of this group are not essentially different from other parents, nor was it felt that the temperamental characteristics in the infants were caused by the parents, but rather that the care of these infants made demands on the parents for firm, patient, consistent and tolerant handling, so that these children, in fact, high-lighted the parental reaction to stress. These observations, therefore, lead us to examine the child's nurture.

NURTURE

In the developing child, this comprises his immediate environment, usually home and later also school, and the influences of the wider community in which he lives.

The child's great need is for security, and whilst it may be helpful for illustration to examine the child's material environment, cultural environment and emotional environment, each of these areas makes some impact on the others.

The material environment

The degree of affluence or poverty to which a child is exposed during his early years will influence his future standards in many ways. In times of relative prosperity, parental affection may be shown by over-indulgence with material gifts. The child from a poor home may be unable to join in school trips or other extra-curricular activities, for financial reasons. He may feel discriminated against because of poor clothing, or free school meals. (Perhaps there is something to be said for school uniform!) The present increase in redundancies, unemployment and short time working is a reminder of periods, earlier in our history, when the problem of material deprivation loomed large for all except the privileged few. With improved housing, clothing, food, education, and the control of infection, the focus of emphasis in recent decades has moved from material deprivation to cultural deprivation and emotional deprivation. However, the work of Dr. Harriet Wilson in her 'Seaport' study, *Delinquency and Child Neglect*, the Newsons' studies in Nottingham and the report published in 1970 by Robert Holman and his colleagues, *Socially Deprived Families in Britain*, draw attention to that new social class, the underprivileged, and underline the serious degree of material deprivation which still exists in this country. Whilst admitting that many material problems have their origin in the emotional difficulties of the parents, one cannot help wondering if emotional deprivation has been over-emphasised to the neglect or the tremendous material handicaps of some families. Many highly-intelligent people would find themselves stretched, if they had to budget for their families on the allowance to which they would be entitled on Social Security. Those existing on these allowances often belong to that section of the community which is least well-endowed intellectually and their energy may be sapped by serious physical ill-health. Many professional mothers find life demanding when they combine a job with running a home, even when regular daily domestic help is available, but it is just this same daily domestic help who has to return to her home and face up to her family's demands at the end of the day, without the aid of the washing machine, electric mixer, etc., which eases life for the professional working-mother. If there is adequate space in the home, the mother overwhelmed by a noisy brood can gain peace and quiet in another area of the house, but for the less fortunate, there may be but one living room with multi-occupancy in the bedrooms.

The cultural environment
Where parents marry and remain within their own community, they have an awareness of the behavioural expectations of that community. This knowledge may contribute to their basic emotional security. The expectancy of the culture in which a child grows up can have a profound effect on his development, as he may be required to conform to the behaviour demanded from a particular culture or social class. Recently we have been made aware of this, by the increasing mobility within our society and the pattern of immigration.

The number of immigrant children arriving in this country demonstrates some of the problems which a change of culture can create and, for example, many Asian teenage girls who have completed their education in this country and seen their Western friends choosing their own fiancés, resent their parent's insistence on an arranged marriage. The problem of mixed marriage, be it a mixture of race or religion, can create distress for teenagers and parents alike and may become the focus for aggressive feelings. The use of corporal punishment in the upbringing of children, both at home and at school, is less common in this country today than earlier in the century, but for non-indigenous children parents may still use the rod. Offspring of such parents may feel 'hard done by', compared with their schoolmates. It is important that those working with disturbed teenagers should be aware of, and have a respect for, cultural backgrounds of non-indigenous groups.

The Newsons have described the British middle class as the 'epic of postponed pleasure'. Children of middle-class parents are encouraged to defer gratification of their demands, to save for, and earn their reward. Middle-class parents tend to adopt child-centred methods when bringing up their offspring and these parents are more likely to withdraw affection in order to show displeasure, resulting in strong conscience-formation. For the less privileged sections of the community, there is often considerable uncertainty about the future and procrastination can be dangerous, so that one learns to live for the moment, with immediate gratification of desire. Professional parents are less likely to adopt physical methods of punishment and aggressive behaviour amongst the children themselves is tolerated less readily.

Cultural stimulation in the middle-class home contrasts with the cultural deprivation of the less prosperous. Where money for basic essentials such as food, clothing and furnishings is limited, there will be no surplus for a daily paper, books or even jigsaws, crayons, pencils and paper, which would not even have to be requested in a more affluent home. Parents who are worn down by the concerns of everyday living, have not the time or energy to spend with their children in leisure pursuits, or supervising homework. The middle-class child has the advantage of commencing school with an awareness of the teacher's expectation of him, as the teacher will usually have come from a similar background, whereas the child from the working class home has first to come to terms with the teacher. For these children, school can be a frustrating experience and this is discussed further in the chapter on non-attendance at school.

As we are increasingly being made aware in our society, cultural influences affect attitudes towards children of different sex. Aggressive play amongst boys is acceptable and may even be encouraged, whereas the tomboyish girl is discouraged. It will be interesting to see what changes may emerge, as the emphasis on sexual equality continues.

The emotional environment

As we have become aware of the basic essentials for physical health such as housing, sanitation and nutrition, so it is recognised that certain necessities are equally required for emotional well-being. These are:

1. Emotional security.
2. Love, acceptance and respect for the developing child.
3. The opportunity for the child to make sustained relationships.
4. Clearly defined and consistently enforced limits.

1. Emotional security

In a sense, emotional security is the sum of the succeeding requirements, and the loved and respected child, who has been able to make sustained relationships and to develop self-imposed behavioural controls, is likely to become the mature adult with appropriate self-esteem and is less likely to present with a major emotional problem in adolescence.

2. Respect for the child

Ideally, each child should be a wanted child, should be encouraged to make the best use of his attributes, free from comparison with other members of the family of the same or an earlier generation. His development can be helped by parental awareness of the behaviour to be expected and the needs associated with each age. Just as one would not expect an infant to walk and talk, so one would not expect a toddler to distinguish between right and left. Temper tantrums, accepted at the toddler stage, may become a cause for concern if persisting in to the early teens. Increasing responsibility, according to the child's level of maturity, is valuable preparation for the later demands of adolescence. Overall, however, the need for security is paramount and each child needs to be valued for himself.

Initially, the emotional environment is provided by the home and by the parents or substitute parents. The key to parental attitudes may be tied up in events which ante-date the child's conception. Many parents work out problems from their own childhood through their offspring and endeavour to ensure that a particular area of frustration, which made an impact on their life, is not a problem for their child. For example, the parent, who grew up in an orphanage and considers that he had a deprived childhood, is sometimes unable to deny his child any material demand and yet may have difficulty in meeting his own child's emotional needs; the parent who had an over-strict mother or father will often compensate by being particularly indulgent to his own child; the parent who was unable to fulfil his academic ambitions may have a high level of academic aspiration for his offspring, regardless of the child's intellectual capabilities. If a marriage resulting from the conception of a child proves to be unsatisfactory, or if the child is conceived in the emotional aftermath of a parental reconciliation following a period of separation, the child may be treated, or maltreated, as special. Similarly, the child, who is conceived to replace a sibling (brother or sister) who has died, possibly in tragic circumstances, may have a role thrust upon him; he is likely to be a particularly precious chiid. These are a few examples of the way in which parental attitudes towards, and expectancy for, a given child may influence the emotional atmosphere in which a child grows up, and may interfere with the child's capacity to function as an individual in his own right.

Lone parent families are providing the nurture for an increasing number of children, and these have their own material and emotional problems, which will be considered further in the next section.

3. Sustained relationships

The family is all important for the developing child. Here he is cared for in his early days of dependency, and through the physical care which he receives, there is also communication at an emotional level, so that the child forms an attachment or emotional bond with the persons caring for him. In a conventional, nuclear family he will have contact with an adult male and an adult female, and from these initial attachments it is thought that the basis for future inter-personal relationships is laid. A harmonious home adds immeasurably to the child's security and provides him with a satisfactory model of each sex to emulate.

No one can replace good parents, especially the mother, but sometimes, owing to unavoidable factors, such as illness of the parent or child, or death of a parent, substitute care has to be provided. Ideally, this is provided in the child's home environment, so that he only has to adjust to the change of adult caring for him and does not have to adapt to strange circumstances. Often a familiar relative may be able to help out at times of crisis, but for some families this may not be feasible and extra-familial help has to be found. A home-help or visiting house-mother may be available from the Local Authority, but in certain circumstances a child may have to be taken into the care of the Local Authority or a voluntary children's nursery or home.

Parental absence and illness Breaks in the parent–child relationship may arise from a variety of reasons, with a tendency to contribute to emotional problems in the child. The reasons for parental absence have recently been examined in considerable detail, and will certainly deserve further study. *Death* of a parent may be sudden, or may have been preceded by a shorter or longer period of ill health. Following the death, the surviving parent's grief may mean that he or she may be unable to meet the child's emotional needs. There is evidence that the death of a parent may be associated with psychiatric disturbance in the child, and, even where the death occurred earlier in the child's life, emotional symptoms are more likely to develop in adolescence than at the time of the bereavement. The social consequences of the bereavement may also be important.

Professor Michael Rutter, in his monograph *Children of Sick Parents* has shown that *parental illness*, be it physical or psychiatric, has a deleterious effect on developing children, particularly if the child is in any way involved with the symptomatology, as when a mother has a psychiatric illness. This last observation has been confirmed by a further study undertaken by a psychologist in Birmingham (Mr. Graham Jones), who has also found reason to be concerned about the adequacy of the substitute care available.

The present emphasis on the community care of the mentally ill, which is allied to recurring admissions to psychiatric hospitals, alternating with periods of residence in the community, when the psychiatrically ill individual has a period of remission, means that those patients who are married now return to their families. Children find it difficult to adjust to the alterations in a parent's mental state and may present with emotional symptoms, so that at times it seems as if parental return to the community results in their children being taken into the care of the Local Authority, or arrangements made for boarding school placement.

However, more serious to the security of the developing child is the *broken home* and, more particularly, the parental discord which is likely to have preceded the break-up of the 'marriage'. The child exposed to severe parental disharmony is likely to present with anti-social symptoms. Parental separation may be preferable for the child than continuing exposure to parental scenes, although too often the child's future care may become a bone of contention between the parents, the child being but a puppet in legal hands (the mass media present all too frequent examples of such situations). The child's allegiance may be split between his parents and this may be an area of strain for him.

Lone parent families are usually the outcome of illegitimacy, parental separation or divorce, or bereavement, thus it is difficult to disentangle the factors contributing to emotional disturbance in children growing up in such a situation. However, certain myths have been exploded so that, for example, the mother rearing a son on her own has no need to be concerned that his masculinity in adult life will be impaired. Nevertheless, children in one parent families suffer from a degree of material deprivation, and have one less parent as an identification model. The key factors relate to the physical and emotional stability of the single parent and the relationships which the child has with this one parent.

Whilst the ideal situation for the developing child is a harmonious, stable home-environment, with both parents, and there is evidence of emotional stress for some children where this is not the case, there is also a group of children whose parents are so rejecting that the parental home is an unhealthy environment and detrimental to their future welfare. Battered babies are, of course, the extreme example in this group. In such a situation, it is essential that, if the child is to have adequate emotional stability, removal from home to foster care or a Local Authority children's home will be required.

It became recognised that children admitted to institutional care suffered from a lack of stimulation and had inadequate opportunity to make sustained relationships with staff. In part, this was due to a poor staff/child ratio, but critical examination of the deployment of staff has shown that if one member of the staff gets a child up, toilets, washes and dresses that child, a relationship can be formed which is not possible if the child is treated by the 'conveyor-belt' system, that is, handed to one member of staff who toilets him on to the next who washes him and then to a third who dresses him, etc. King, Raynes and Tizard have compared the treatment of children in a children's home with those in a long-stay paediatric ward and in a mental-subnormality hospital, to the detriment of the hospital system, where 'conveyor belt' activity tends to be the rule, so that although, for acute short-term care, as on a paediatric ward, it may be expedient for all staff to get to know all the patients, the 'conveyor-belt' type of care is undesirable in the more domestic living situation of the long-stay paediatric ward, childrens' psychiatric ward or children's home.

With the shorter working week, changing staff and unpopularity of weekend working, it is becoming increasingly difficult to provide residential care up to a desired standard and for this and other reasons, there is increasing emphasis on adoption and good foster care. How can one provide adequate individual stimulation for small children in a group situation? For example, it was only when a handicapped four years old boy, living in a residential nursery, had his first weekend with a foster aunt and uncle that it was appreciated that he had not realised that grown-ups went to bed, whereas most parents wish that their offspring would stay out of parental bed in the early hours of the morning!

As a result of modern methods of medical treatment, children require in-patient hospital treatment less frequently and admissions are of shorter duration than formerly. One of the outcomes of work on maternal deprivation has been a better understanding of the effects of admission to hospital on the child, so that in many children's wards continuous visiting is acceptable. Adult hospitals, however, seem to be less aware of the effect of parent-child separation, though in the more enlightened hospitals, children under 14 are being allowed to visit sick parents for a short time during a prolonged admission. There is, however, another side to continuous visiting of children in hospital. Recently, the author has come across a number of children who have not been in hospital themselves, but whose sibling has had a prolonged stay as an in-patient. The child in hospital has, in some instances, died, but even where this has not been the case, the ill child does not appear to have suffered any emotional ill effects as a result of the separation, whereas the child at home has been deprived, since he has been looked after by whoever would have him, for many hours at a time, and has suffered a partial rejection when the parents have been under stress.

4. Limit setting

In order to conform to the demands of Western society, parents have to teach their children to accept some limits on their behaviour. Many studies have been made on how this can be achieved. It is generally accepted that inconsistent and erratic discipline is more harmful than too little or too much discipline. But perhaps it is surprising how wide a range of degree of severity or laxity, or indeed method of discipline used, is tolerated by the average child without any obvious ill effects. Rather, it seems that

the key may lie in the parent–child relationship, which is all important, and if this is good and the child respects, and is respected by,
his parent, the outcome is satisfactory. Where the parent–child
relationship is unsatisfactory and the parent is rejecting or hostile
towards the child, there may be frequent punishment and there is
evidence to suggest that this may have undesirable repercussions
for the child's future behaviour.

Studies of discipline in the home have been closely allied to
examination of parental attitudes. Two dimensions of parental attitudes have emerged from these studies. First of all, parents may
be rated at one end of a scale in terms of their warmth and acceptance of a child. This is usually associated with child-centred child
rearing practices; at the other end of this scale, is parental rejection,
manifested by hostility and aggression towards the child. The second dimension examines the degree of control exercised, extending
from restrictiveness and parental autocracy at one end, to permissiveness at the other hand (N.B. the phrase over-permissive has
not been used). Within these two dimensions, four combinations
are possible:

1. The accepting, permissive parent.
2. The accepting, restrictive parent.
3. The rejecting, permissive parent.
4. The rejecting, restrictive parent.

The accepting, permissive parent has been regarded as the
nearest to the ideal parent and the progeny from this background
tend to be confident children, with high self-esteem, who are
accepted by their contemporaries as friends and leaders.

The accepting, restrictive regime, results in children who are
more dependent and more conforming, who also find it more
difficult to make friends.

Rejecting, restrictive parents produce aggressive children who
are too cowed to express their hostility directly and so take it out
indirectly, towards their peer group, or internalise it on themselves,
whereas the aggressive feelings of the offspring of rejecting, permissive parents are expressed more directly.

Parental attitudes are difficult to examine objectively and it may
be that children with different temperaments respond better to one

kind of parental regime than another. Obviously, a lot more work
has still to be done in this area.

From the foregoing it will be seen that the individual approaching adolescence has been moulded by many factors, from
conception through the first decade of life. We are now in a position
to examine the developmental task of the adolescent.

REFERENCES AND FURTHER READING

Coopersmith, S. *The Antecedents of Self Esteem.* W. H. Freeman and
  Co., 1967.
Holman, R., Lafitte, F., Spencer, K. and Wilson, H. *Socially Deprived
  Families in Britain.* Bedford Square Press, 1970.
Jones, Graham. *Personal Communication.*
King, R. D., Tizard, J. and Raynes, N. V. *Patterns of Residential Care:
  Sociological Studies of Institutions for Handicapped Children.*
  Routledge and Kegan Paul, 1971.
Lilienfeld, A. M. and Pasamanick, B. 'The Association of Maternal and
  Fetal Factors with the Development of Cerebral Palsy and Epilepsy.'
  American Journal Obstet. Gynec., 1955, 70, 93.
Mussen, P. H., Conger, J. J. and Kagan, J. *Child Development and Per-
  sonality.* Harper & Row, London, 4th Edition, 1974.
Neligan, G. A. 'Late Sequelae of Pre-Natal Complication.' British Jour-
  nal of Hospital Medicine, 1970, 3, 587.
Newson, J. and Newson, E. *Patterns of Infant Care in an Urban Com-
  munity.* Allen & Unwin Ltd., 1963. Penguin Books, 1965.
Newson, J. and Newson, E. *Four Years Old in an Urban Community.*
  Allen & Unwin Ltd., 1968. Penguin Books, 1970.
Pasamanick, B., Rogers, M. E. and Lilienfeld, A. M. 'Pregnancy
  Experience and the Development of Behaviour Disorders in Children.'
  American Journal of Psychiatry, 1956, 112, 613.
Ratcliffe, F. G., Stewart, A. L., Melville, M. M., Jacobs, P. A. and Peay,
  A. J. 'Chromosome Studies of 3,500 New-born Male Infants.' Lancet,
  1970, 1, 121.
Rutter, M. *Children of Sick Parents: An Environmental and Psychiatric
  Study.* Institute of Psychiatry. Maudsley Monograph No. 16. Oxford
  University Press, 1966.
Rutter, M. *Maternal Deprivation Reassessed.* Penguin Books, 1972.
Thomas, A., Chess, S., Birch, H. and Hertzig, M. A Longitudinal Study
  of Primary Reaction Patterns in Children.' Comprehensive Psychiatry,
  1960, 1, 103.
Wilson, H. *Delinquency and Child Neglect.* Allen & Unwin Ltd., 1962.
*Wolff, S. *Children Under Stress.* Allen Lane The Penguin Press, 1969.

Recommended selected reading.

2 The developmental task of adolescence

Adolesence is derived from the Latin *adolescere* meaning to grow. It is defined in the *Shorter Oxford English Dictionary* as 'a process or condition of growing up; the period between childhood and maturity extending from fourteen to twenty-five in males and twelve to twenty-one in females'. The term is said to have been used first by Rousseau in 1762.

It is generally accepted that the onset of adolescence is associated with biological sexual maturation and the completion, with psychological maturation. The problem is in recognising these end points and making allowance for considerable individual variation. Some workers use the term adolescence as synonymous with teenage, while others use it for individuals in the second decade of life. For expediency, one imagines that with the raising of the school leaving age to sixteen, planners will make provision for the pre-school child (0 to 4-plus years) the child at the stage of primary education (5 to 11-plus years) then secondary education (11-plus to 16-plus years) and finally young people, including the young school leaver and those who move on to further or tertiary education.

LEGAL ASPECTS OF ADOLESCENCE AND THE AGE OF CONSENT

Some of the underdeveloped countries practice initiation rites, following which the young person is accepted as a responsible member of the community. Some religions and some denominations of the Christian church have similar ceremonies at adolescence, for example, the Jewish Barmitzvah and the Anglican confirmation. On the whole, Western secular society is rather more confused about the age at which individuals can accept responsibility. At the present time, some of the significant ages in England are:

10 years—the age of criminal responsibility.

16 years—from September, 1972 this has become the statutory school leaving age. It is also the age at which an individual can give consent to sexual relations, though he or she can only marry with parental consent. Again, with parental consent the individual can live away from home. He can be offered or sold tobacco.

From the medical point of view, it is important to remember that sixteen is the age of consent to medical treatment. Strictly speaking, a doctor can only see an adolescent's parents with his consent, after the age of 16. There is no doubt that a child committed to the care of the local authority can give his or her consent to medical treatment at the age of 16. There is no law which says that a child under the age of 16 may not give his own consent, and indeed many younger children may consult their family doctor in the absence of a parent and treatment is prescribed. However, if a child under the age of 16 insists on signing himself out of hospital, it is necessary to inform the parent or guardian of the position.

17 years—a teenager can live away from home without parental consent. Up until the age of seventeen court proceedings are usually dealt with by a Juvenile Court.

18 years—now the age of majority. Marriage can take place without parental consent and an individual of this age may buy or consume intoxicating liquor in a public bar, in addition to having voting rights.

ADOLESCENT DEVELOPMENT

Meeting an individual for the first time, one may be struck by his stature, or certain facial characteristics. One may feel that he appears particularly stupid or relatively intelligent. He may be good-tempered, cheerful or rather reserved. By and large, we analyse his attributes under subheadings:

1. Physical
2. Intellectual
3. Emotional

In the same way, it is proposed to use these headings to examine normal adolescent development. It is convenient to look at each area in isolation, although in practice there is some inter-relationship.

Physical growth at adolescence
Physical growth at adolescence includes alteration in hormone production, in the reproductive system, in overall stature and changes in other tissues.

Hormonal changes at adolescence
Hormones are the secretion of certain internal glands known as the endocrine glands. The most important of these at puberty is the pituitary gland, which is situated at the base of the brain, the secretions of which control the cortex of the adrenal glands (which are situated in the abdomen, one above each kidney) and sex organs (testes in the male and ovaries in the female). Before puberty, in boys and girls, small amounts of sex hormones are produced, probably from the adrenal glands. In both sexes there is an increase in androgen production (male sex hormone) at the age of eight to ten, with a much sharper rise at adolescence. From the age of seven, there is also an increase in female sex hormone (oestrogen) production. It is thought that the rise in the production of oestrogens and androgens at adolescence is due to the formation of these hormones by the sex organs (gonads) which are stimulated by gonadotrophin, a hormone secreted in the anterior part of the pituitary gland, but under the ultimate control of that part of the brain known as the hypothalamus. Gonadotrophins are measured by analysing their excretion in twenty-four-hour specimens of urine and are scarcely, if at all, detectable before the beginning of adolescence, but appear about the time the testes begin to enlarge in boys and at the onset of breast development in girls. The

measurement of gonadotrophin excretion is probably the most accurate available method of measuring pubertal development.

At adolescence, oestrogen excretion rises very sharply in girls and becomes cyclical—even when excretion in girls is at its monthly minimum, it is greater than in boys. The oestrogen cycle appears to be established at about the time that the breast buds appear and the spurt in height begins. The values continue to increase until some years after menstruation is established.

Gonadal development in adolescence

In boys, the first sign of impending puberty is usually acceleration of growth of the testes and scrotum. Slight growth of pubic hair may begin at about this time, but it proceeds slowly until commencement of the general growth spurt and from then on pubic hair development proceeds rapidly. The spurt of growth in height begins about a year after testicular growth is apparent, and at this time the penis also begins to enlarge. Usually, the appearance of facial and axillary hair is relatively late, occurring about two years after the first appearance of pubic hair. Enlargement of the larynx is associated with a deepening of the voice, which begins to be noticeable when development of the penis is nearing completion. The male breast undergoes changes, and in about a third of boys there is distinct enlargement of breast-tissue midway through adolescence and this persists for twelve to eighteen months. The first ejaculation is culturally, as well as biologically, determined, and occurs about a year after the beginning of the acceleration in growth of the penis. For the average American boy, this is just under 14. In 90 per cent of a large sample, the age range for first ejaculation was 11–16 years.

In girls, the appearance of breast buds is usually the first sign of puberty, although the appearance of pubic hair may occasionally precede it. As in all aspects of physical development, there is considerable variation with age, and this is particularly true of the menarche (first menstrual period). This tends to occur after the peak of the growth-spurt has occurred. The early menstrual cycles are anovulatory, that is, they are not associated with the release of an ovum and so at this stage, girls are infertile. Maximum fertility occurs in the early- to mid-twenties. There is considerable variation in the age at the first menstrual period and anytime between 11 and

17 years is accepted as being within the normal range. There is some correlation in the age of menarche in mother and daughter and it would appear that there is a genetic influence operating; if a mother had her first period early, her daughter is likely to follow suit. There is also an association between menarche, height and intelligence; taller and more intelligent girls being younger at the menarche.

Although menstruation itself is physical, there are emotional overtones. Some girls are pleased and proud when they start menstruating, while others feel ashamed. In the days when girls did not take part in physical recreation when menstruating, sometimes an otherwise conscientious girl of high moral standards would forge a note for the games-mistress, rather than let her age peers know that she had not yet commenced menstruation.

Growth-spurt in adolescence

This refers particularly to the sudden increase in height and weight which occurs in adolescence. As with other aspects of physical development, there is considerable individual variation. Before adolescence, boys and girls are practically the same height for age. In boys, the growth-spurt occurs between $12\frac{1}{2}$ and 15 years. During this period there is a gain in height of 20 cm (with a range of 10–30 cm) and a gain in weight of 20 kg (with a range of 7–30 kg). The maximum velocity is at 14, but the range is 12 to 17 years. On average, girls have their growth-spurt two years younger than boys—$10\frac{1}{2}$ to 13 years—but the increase in growth is smaller than in boys. The increase in height is related to an increase in length of the trunk, rather than the length of the legs and the ratio of trunk length to leg length increases during adolescence. In boys, every muscle and skeletal dimension takes part in the adolescent growth-spurt and the heart and abdominal organs also increase in size. Clumsiness in adolescence is associated with these changes. Again in boys, there is an increase in red blood cells. Acne, a particularly distressing type of skin rash, occurring on the face and upper part of the trunk, may be prominent during adolescence and cause a great deal of unhappiness on account of its unsightliness.

These, in brief, are the major changes in physical growth at adolescence. It is important to remember that in girls, the changes occur approximately two years earlier than in boys and again there is considerable variation in the age and order in which the changes take place. Most of the work in this area has been carried out by Dr. J. M. Tanner and the reader who would like to know about growth changes in more detail is referred to his book *Growth at Adolescence.*

Psychological effects of puberty
The boy who has an early growth-spurt in adolescence is often at an advantage in comparison with his contemporaries, once he has passed the gangling stage, as, until they catch up with him, his athletic prowess may be noteworthy and this may help him to develop an overall confidence which is to his benefit. Some psychological work has shown that parents, teachers and other adults in the teenager's environment, treat him according to his size: the small adolescent is still treated as a child, whereas the tall youth is given respect more appropriate to his adult stature. One practical example of this is the admission of the under-sized teenager to a children's ward as a matter of expediency. The ward regime will almost certainly be geared to the needs of the prepubertal patient, so that the developing teenager is likely to find himself in an emotionally stunting situation but, in addition, he has sustained a blow to his self-esteem, as a result of chronological misplacement. The same situation can arise in relation to placements throughout the range of Community Homes (the former Children's Homes and Approved Schools).

There is still folklore in existence in relation to menstruation. If a girl stops menstruating there are two possible explanations, first, that she is pregnant and second that the blood, if it does not come out, must go somewhere; not so long ago, it used to be thought that the blood must go to the head. This was based on the shrewd observation that people who are emotionally disturbed may have an associated amenorrhoea. The deduction was that it must be the amenorrhoea, that is, the cessation of the menstrual flow, which caused the emotional upset, but we know now that although the observation was correct, the deduction was wrong and usually the amenorrhoea is secondary to the psychiatric illness. Similarly, young girls leaving home for the first time, to become resident in nurses' homes, halls of residence or domestic service, commonly have irregular menstruation, often with prolonged periods of amenorrhoea. It is now thought that the amenorrhoea is due to the emotional upheaval and is mediated through the part of the brain known as the hypothalamus. With increasing emancipation of women, perhaps less close chaperonage, and more co-education in schools, girls seem to cope better with alterations in their environment, with less menstrual upset.

Intellectual development in adolescence

Piaget has suggested that, in the second decade of life, there is an alteration in the type of thinking and whereas, formerly, the child has thought in concrete terms, as he approaches puberty he learns to think more abstractly. Surprisingly little has been done to examine this concept, but some recent work by Professor Peel of the Education Department, University of Birmingham, tends to support Piaget's views, although it would appear that the development of concept-formation has not been acquired even by all honours graduates, on the tests which Professor Peel has devised!

J. W. B. Douglas and his colleagues took a sample of children born in this country in the first week in March, 1946 and followed them up at regular intervals. They showed that in their attainments in the early stages of their development, girls tended to be ahead of boys matched for equal intelligence. For example, girls learn to talk and read earlier than boys. Boys lag behind in their attainments until puberty, but after their growth-spurt they tend to improve on their attainments and from then on they achieve more than girls of equal intelligence.

Emotional development in adolescence

The emotional tasks of adolescence can be conveniently seen as:

1. The attainment of a sexual identity through stages of psycho-sexual development.
2. The attainment of separation and independence from parents, with a return to parents in a new relationship, based on relative equality.
3. Development of a personal moral-value system.
4. Career choice.

These are no mean tasks yet, interestingly, the majority of adolescents achieve these goals with little disruption. Throughout this period, the adolescent will remain an idealist. He sees things in terms of black and white and is reluctant to accept the shades of grey.

Psycho-sexual development

The first sign of psycho-sexual arousal may be a homosexual 'crush' involving a person of the same sex. This phase appears to be more common amongst girls than boys and occurs more noticeably in closed communities. Teachers moving from a girls' day school to a girls' boarding-school are often struck by the greater problem in the residential setting. It seems that this phase is less marked than formerly, presumably influenced by cultural change and again by the increase in co-educational schooling, lessening chaperonage and changes in the social setting. When it does occur, it rarely presents a problem if the adult can cope with the situation. Understandably, he or she cannot help being flattered by this hero-worship and the more insecure adult may reciprocate at a social level. Subsequently, this friendship may prove embarrassing for the adult, who will attempt to withdraw him or herself from the teenager. Teenagers feel intensely and in a rejecting situation such as this they are 'heartbroken'. Occasionally, suicidal attempts may result from such circumstances. The ideal situation is the one in which the adult is unaware of the teenager's feelings and is worshipped from afar, the teenager's day being made by acknowledgment of her presence by the significant adult.

The next stage is that of the heterosexual 'crush'. This again usually involves an older person. A study of romantic literature would suggest that at the beginning of this century, a clergyman was usually the object of a teenager's fantasy life, to be ousted by film stars and now by pop stars and well-known footballers. Pin-ups of the favoured ones are common wall coverings in teenage bedrooms. Occasionally, an older adult who is in the teenager's immediate environment may be the recipient of favour. Rarely, this may develop into a physical sexual relationship and, occasionally, the outcome may be an extra-marital pregnancy.

After this, heterosexual interest tends to drop down the age range, and one sees groups of boys and girls of similar age joining in activities together. Double-dating is a relatively common way of reducing a teenager's anxiety on his first date. Gradually, there is pairing off and frequent changes of partner are not uncommon at this stage. Again, the adolescent's intensity of feeling becomes important, and the loss of face when a friendship breaks off may provoke a crisis and even a suicidal attempt.

Teenagers tend to find the current heterosexual relationship all-absorbing, so that in many instances all social contact revolves around the boy-friend of the moment. When the pair splits up, the teenager may not only lose a boy-friend, but find herself in a situation of relative social isolation, and require family support to become involved again in group leisure activities. Fortunately, although feelings are intense, they are not long-lasting and in most instances the arrival of a new boy-friend soothes the wounded pride.

I have described the various stages of psychosexual development as though a given individual would pass through them all, but this is not necessarily so and, indeed, would be the exception rather than the rule. However, it is easier to describe psychosexual development in this way for the purposes of demonstration.

There are considerable differences in the expectations from a heterosexual relationship when looked at from the viewpoint of a boy or a girl. Whilst, for a boy, the physical gratification of his sex urge is paramount, many girls are able to sublimate their sexual feelings and regard the relationship, with promise of future security, as important. To what extent this differences in attitude is biological, or is related to what may be regarded as more intensive conditioning of girls during their earlier years, remains to be seen. There must be few girls whose parents have not indicated the vulnerability associated with fertility and that, literally as well as metaphorically, it is the girl who is left 'holding the baby'. Perhaps it is surprising that more adults are not sexually maladjusted, considering the emphasis on inhibition of sexual responses to which they have been exposed in our culture, during childhood and adolescence.

The adolescent's adjustment to his sexual role appears to be closely related to his relationship with his parents and particularly the same-sex parent. The interaction of biological and psychological factors is considered further in Chapter 15.

Attainment of separation and independence from parents
Just as the young child learns to walk in the second year of life and

by the time he commences school has become relatively independent physically, so the hallmark of adolescence is the attainment of
emotional independence. The individual who enters the adolescent
period of life from a stable background, with reasonably good self-
esteem, will cope with the drive towards independence. For the insecure youngster, the path can be rough. Parental awareness of the
need for the individual teenager to 'stand on his own feet' is important. With insight, many parents recognise when their adolescent
offspring is ready to accept more responsibility and when he needs
to have pressures reduced. The fact that a teenager no longer needs
to confide in them is regarded by some parents as hurtful, whereas
the reverse is true, and it is often indicative of the teenager's ability
to cope with the demands of adolescence. The term 'generation
gap' has become a cliché, but for some it seems to be an essential
phase of development on the way to mature adulthood, which is
characterised by the acceptance of *interdependence*, so that the
developing youngster can return to the parents in a new
relationship, based on relative equality.

As mentioned earlier, many cultures indicate to the developing
teenager the point at which they may accept further responsibility,
but in secular society in this country it is less clear. For many
children, they become adult when they become breadwinners, yet it
is the teenager who is best-endowed physically and intellectually
who may continue in further education and thus to some degree remain financially dependent on his parents until well into the third
decade of life. On the other hand, those teenagers who are
employed may be recognised to have larger amounts of uncom-
mitted money than any other section of the community and the
leisure-industry is keenly aware of this.

As the infant was weaned in the first year of life, so the adolescent requires a period of emotional weaning. The majority of
parents gradually give their children increasing responsibility, initially in material things, for example, choosing their own clothes,
spending their pocket money and then, bit-by-bit, allowing them to
accept responsibility in more important areas of life and helping
them to develop a system of moral values. However, those parents
who had difficulty in emancipation during their own adolescence,
may have difficulty in allowing their offspring to have independence
in certain ways.

Commonly, we talk of 'cutting the apron-strings' and as il-lustrating the striving towards independence, this analogy is useful. The apron-string may be cut by the parent or the teenager and equally the parent or the adolescent may retie the knot. Sometimes, one comes across a parent who feels that a youth ought to be less dependent and should move into the community. Such a parent may hint that he ought to be more involved with teenage parties or with the opposite sex. Usually, the adolescent is only too well aware of the situation, realising that he is not 'with it', is uncertain of himself and is unsure what steps to take in order to become in-volved. If and when he succeeds in getting an invitation to a teenage party, his self-consciousness is heightened by the memory of parental comment on his difficulties. This is an example of the parent who attempts to cut the knot before the teenager is ready.

Another parent is the one who undermines what little confidence a teenager has and is reluctant to let him venture into a given situa-tion, in case it should get out of hand, even though this is unlikely to happen. Often a youth has to rebel to break away from this situation and this, in particular, is a time when the psychiatrist may become involved directly. In the most extreme cases of this type, the teenager may require in-patient psychiatric treatment in a hospital adolescent unit. One of our more technical terms for this is the so-called 'hostile-dependent relationship', when a teenager reacts with marked hostility to his dependence on a parent. Often this relationship is almost parasitic; a parent, or often both parents, fostering a child's dependence on the home. A normally confor-ming, clinging child often shows a surprising degree of aggression, both verbal and physical in such a situation.

The youngster who cuts the apron-string often seems to be a well-adjusted teenager who can move forward on his own, but oc-cassionally he may be too self-confident and get himself into situations with which he cannot cope. On some of these occassions, he may come into conflict with the law. Teenage rebellion may be healthy and draw attention to emotional difficulties, but occasional-ly it may recoil on the individual.

The teenager who is continually re-tying the knot in the apron-string has been described to some extent in an earlier paragraph and there is usually a reciprocal relationship with one of the parents, although occasionally this is not the case.

Ideally, however, rather than cutting the apron-string, one would like to think that it could be left loose, so that although rarely taut it could be shortened at moments of crisis by the parent or the adolescent.

It seems as if each generation of teenagers is helped to move from dependence towards independence through establishing increasing relationships with its peer group. The reader will be familiar with teenage gangs, teddy-boys, mods and rockers, hippies, skinheads and greasers. Each group was recognised by a specific 'uniform' and this has included distinctive hairstyles. Unfortunately, more than an outward and visible sign has been necessary latterly and, in the last decade, one of the ways of teenage identification has been misuse of drugs. Adolescents test out ideas, opinions and activities through their peer group. An idea which has been discussed with an adult is tried out at a coffee bar or other meeting place and, if approved by his contemporaries, the adolescent's confidence is boosted. However, if they frown on the idea, he will admit that it originally came from an adult and that he was testing out the situation with his friends, fully aware that they would disapprove—an example of a face-saving ruse.

It is at this stage that popularity with contemporaries is important to adolescents. Those teenagers who have difficulty in forming such relationships may lose valuable support at this time in their development. Many parents feel threatened by the adolescent's peer group, as they feel unable to understand the rapidly changing fashions, interests and vocabularies with which they come in contact. At times, parents and peer groups may be in a situation of rivalry, but often each seeks the same goals. Even those adolescents who are fully accepted by their contemporaries have moments of intense loneliness and self-doubt. The unpopular adolescent has a great additional burden to carry.

During this period of emotional growth, the adolescent spends a lot of time in self-analysis, liking or disliking what he sees. He may be conscious of a gap between the self that he is at present and the mature person he would like to be. At this stage, teenagers may cast themselves in various roles and try out different ways of coping with life. An awareness of this behaviour may appear to the youngster as insincerity, as he is unsure which is his real self. Feelings like this, and heightened self-consciousness, can be difficult to live with and may contribute to adolescent depression.

Development of a personal moral value system

Tied up with the adolescent's search for an identity is a need to work out where he stands in terms of moral values. In the first decade of life, the youngster is exposed to the parental value system and that of the culture in which he is growing up. As he proceeds through the second decade of life, he has either to incorporate these standards into his own life-style or reject them. Obvious examples in this area relate to religion, drugs and sex before marriage. Adults can argue the pros and cons with the teenager, but in the last analysis, each individual has to make his own decision.

The youth, who rejects the use of alcohol on the grounds that he wants to drive and is not prepared to endanger his life by drinking and driving, will often be respected by his contemporaries, even if they do not accept his views; the teenage son, growing up in a teetotal family, who does not drink because 'my mummy would not like it' will be the object of ridicule, as he has yet to come to terms with the situation for himself. Some teenagers may accompany a parent to church to please the parent, aware that they have no strongly held religious views of their own, but at least they are being honest with themselves. (For other adolescents, the social support of an active church group may be an important prop as they move towards independence.)

It is important that parents should respect the decisions of their off-spring, even if they cannot agree with them.

Sadly, the adolescent has to recognise that the world in which he lives does not practise what is preached. Increasingly, in the school situation the teenager is taught to value himself as a person, but on moving into the world of industry he may find himself but another cog in the machine. Unless he can find satisfaction in his leisure pursuits, he may find it difficult to come to terms with his sphere of employment.

Career choice

In our culture, it is expected that on leaving school, or after a period of further education, a young person will move into paid employment, and a sign of maturity is a commitment to work. The teenager who knows the career he would like to follow has a goal at which to aim and, even if this is not attained, it may provide a focus of stability during a period of turmoil. Should it be attainable, it contributes immensely to the teenager's security and self-esteem. Increasingly, career-guidance is available in schools, but in certain areas the problem may be unemployment rather than indecision on a career choice.

Those involved with adolescents must have an awareness of the developmental needs of the growing teenager and make provision, so that there is space for development in all areas. Adults, who have themselves come to terms with their own areas of strength and weakness, have a liking for youth and a sensitivity to the needs of the maturing youngster, are often in the best position to help those adolescents who get into difficulties. Some of these difficulties are taken up in the next section.

REFERENCES AND FURTHER READING

Douglas, J. W. B. 'Age of Puberty related to Education Ability, Attainment and School Leaving Age.' Journal of Child Psychol. and Psychiat., 1964, 5, 185.

H.M.S.O. (1967). *Report of the Committee of the Age of Majority.* Cmnd. 3342 (Latey report).

*Mussen, P. H., Conger, J. J. and Kagen, J. *Child Development and Personality.* Harper & Row, London, 4th Edition, 1974.

*Pomeroy, Wardell, B. *Boys and Sex.* Delacorte Press, 1968. Pelican Books, 1970.

*Pomeroy, Wardell B. *Girls and Sex.* Delacorte Press, 1969. Pelican Books, 1971.

Peel, E. A. *Postgraduate Lecture*, Hollymoor Hospital, March, 1973.

*Schofield, M. *The Sexual Behaviour of Young People.* Longmans, 1965. Pelican Books, 1968.

Tanner, J. M. *Growth at Adolescence.* Blackwell Scientific Publications Ltd., 2nd Edition, 1962.

Recommended selected reading.

PART 2
DEVIATION IN ADOLESCENCE

3 Presentation, classification, diagnosis and epidemiology in adolescent psychiatry

MODE OF PRESENTATION

The vast majority of adolescents come to terms with their physical development, psycho-sexual development and drive for independence, but there has always been a minority whose disturbed behaviour has presented a challenge to each generation. These young people who find difficulty in meeting the demands of adolescence may present in a variety of ways, but usually come to attention because someone in their environment is concerned about their behaviour. Resulting from this concern, an approach may be made to one of several agencies in the community. For example, when a parent is concerned because a teenager is moody or tearful, the family doctor may be consulted. If there is anxiety because a daughter is coming in late at night, or a youth is defiant, an approach may be made to the local authority Social Service Department. (In April, 1970 the local authority Mental Health, Welfare and Children's Departments amalgamated to form the new local authority Department of Social Services.) Alternatively, an approach may be made to a probation officer or a voluntary agency, such as the Samaritans, the Open Door, or other voluntary counselling service. Occasionally, a parent may make direct contact with a Child Guidance Clinic (*see* below).

If a school is concerned about a pupil's behaviour, or lack of progress, the head teacher may arrange to see the parents and may initiate referral to a Child Guidance Clinic, or advise the parents to consult the family doctor or school medical officer. Nowadays, some schools have a school counsellor, usually a teacher who has had special training in emotional problems of school children.

On the other hand, the earliest indication of behavioural disturbance may be outside the home and school, and the police may be involved and, through them, the probation officer or local authority social worker and later the Juvenile Court.

From any of these sources a psychiatric opinion may be requested, although in many instances the request would be channelled through the family doctor. Indeed, if at all possible, the family doctor should be involved, as he knows many details of the teenager's medical history and what, if any, medication he may be having.

In seeking help, a teenager and his family are likely to make contact with one or more professional workers in a treatment team. Most commonly the team would include:

1. A *psychiatrist*—a doctor who has undertaken an undergraduate course in medicine and who would have spent at least one year as a house doctor at a general hospital before deciding to specialise in psychiatry. The word 'psychiatrist' is derived from the Greek *psyche* meaning mind and *iatros* meaning doctor, so that the psychiatrist specialises in diseases of the mind, just as the cardiologist specialises in diseases of the heart, and the gastro-enterologist in diseases of the alimentary tract. The psychiatrist tends to be asked to see patients who present with disturbed behaviour. Some undertake work with children, others with adults. At present, under the National Health Service, adult psychiatrists tend to be based in hospitals, having beds at a mental hospital or at one of the new psychiatric units in a District General Hospital. Most psychiatrists have out-patient clinics at general hospitals, but under certain circumstances, the family doctor may arrange for a patient to be seen by a specialist in his own home. Child psychiatrists may work similarly to their adult colleagues, or they may work in a special child psychiatric clinic or be based at a local authority Child Guidance Clinic. (Since the 1st April, 1974 some of the Child Guidance Clinics have been taken over by the Area Health Authorities.)

2. A *psychologist* will have taken an Honours Degree in Psychology in a faculty of arts or science and will then have specialised, so that, for example, there is the educational psychologist who works for the local authority Education Department in schools and Child Guidance Clinics, the clinical psychologist who is employed in the National Health Service, particularly in psychiatric units, and the occupational psychologist, who works in industry. Psychology also derives from Greek, *psyche* meaning mind and *logos* meaning knowledge (of the mind), so that he specialises in understanding human behaviour. At one time, the psychologist was thought to be more involved in dealing with normal functioning, leaving deviant functioning to the psychiatrist, but this distinction is no longer applicable.

3. Another key member of the therapeutic team is the *social worker*. Many social workers will have a university degree or college diploma, usually in arts or social science, and will then have undertaken a postgraduate social work qualification. Just as psychologists and doctors specialise, so in the past Social Workers could specialise in child care, when they were known as Child Care Officers; in general hospitals, when they were known as Almoners (later Medical Social Workers); or Mental Health when they were known as Psychiatric Social Workers or Mental Welfare Officers. Probation officers also have an independent post-graduate training. More recently, social work training has become generic, that is, like the medical student, trainees are now learning about all aspects of emotional health, from childhood through to old age, and in relation to physical and mental health. Some social workers continue to work in hospitals and Child Guidance Clinics but the vast majority of social workers are employed by a local authority Department of Social Services.

The clinic

The therapeutic team working with the younger age group is often based in a Child Guidance Clinic, which is usually under the auspices of the local authority. The first Child Guidance clinic in England was opened in 1927. This was a voluntary clinic started by the Jewish Health Organisation in the East End of London. Initially, it was considered that the work of such clinics would be educational and social rather than medical, but, as they developed, there was some confusion over the roles of the members of the teams. The situation was examined by the Underwood Committee which recommended the setting up of joint clinics, their social workers, psychologists and secretarial staff being employed by the local authority and the psychiatrist by the National Health Service. The demand for consultations was greater than the amount of professional time available and this situation continues to the present day, so that lengthy waiting lists have become unavoidable. In order to assess the degree of urgency of each individual referral, some preliminary screening may be done by the social worker or psychologist. A brief interview may be offered to the parent and it can be ascertained at this which team worker would be the most appropriate person to undertake the initial detailed assessment.

Although, theoretically, the services of a Child Guidance Clinic are available until the age of eighteen, on account of its link with the local Education Authority the majority of patients seen at these clinics are of school age and less use has been made of this service by the pre-school child and the young school-leaver. One factor probably contributes particularly to the under-usage of the Child Guidance facilities by the older adolescent. At the clinic, the younger child is encouraged to express his feelings through play, drawings and creative activities; inevitably this includes the use of dolls, doll's houses, and other toys and the more sensitive and insecure adolescent feels threatened at being surrounded by such objects, which he regards himself as having outgrown. Despite the lack of use of these clinics by adolescents, a good Child Guidance Clinic is an example of the high level of community care which can be developed. Many have particularly close links with schools in their area.

In principle, patients are referred to hospital by their family doctors and he refers patients to psychiatric clinics, just as he does to clinics for treatment of physical illness. In practice, a social worker or head teacher may express concern about a patient and advise the family to contact their doctor and thus indirectly instigate a referral to a hospital psychiatric clinic. At times, in hospital clinics, the availability of social workers and (clinical) psychologists may be limited, and in general the team approach has been less well developed. On the other hand, waiting lists are likely to be shorter than at a Child Guidance Clinic and there is usually a close link with the paediatric department of the hospital.

The case history

At the hospital adolescent clinic, the teenager will be seen by the psychiatrist who obtains information from the patient about the present difficulties as seen by him or her. In addition, he will enquire about the family environment, academic and social factors in the school and, if appropriate, the work setting, previous illnesses and overall development. An almost identical case history may be taken from the parents by the social worker whilst the psychiatrist is seeing the teenager or, alternatively, the psychiatrist may take the history from the parents after seeing the adolescent concerned.

If someone goes to his doctor and says he has collapsed with pain in his chest and left arm, in many instances the doctor could make the correct diagnosis of a heart attack before examining him, *i.e.*, the diagnosis is made on the basis of the history alone and no physical signs have to be elicited. There are other examples of this in the field of general medicine and surgery and, occasionally, also in psychiatry, but just as the general physician usually has to elicit physical signs, so the psychiatrist carries out what we call an examination of the patient's mental state and for this it is essential to spend a reasonable amount of time with the patient. This is really the most important part of the psychiatrist's examination. Throughout the interview, the psychiatrist observes the patient's attitude and behaviour. Whilst listening to the patient's account of his difficulties and description of family background, the psychiatrist is also noting the rate at which he is talking, the relevance of his conversation, and any abnormal features which may be apparent. He asks the patient about his mood and attempts to assess it objectively. He enquires about the difficulties the patient may have in thinking and asks special questions in order to elicit such difficulties. He examines the patient's memory and assesses his attention, concentration and what is called his orientation, that is, the patient's awareness of his surroundings, who he is, where he is and when it is, *i.e.*, the date, place and time. The psychiatrist may also make a subjective judgment of the patient's intellectual level, but if necessary this will be followed up with a more objective assessment by a psychologist.

These last areas of examination—orientation, memory, concentration and intelligence are termed the patient's *cognitive* function. If a patient shows disturbance in this area it is most likely that he is suffering from an *organic illness*, that is, the symptoms with which he is presenting have a physical basis.

If the main area of disturbance is of *mood*, for example, marked depression, elation or anxiety, a diagnosis of an *affective illness* is most likely.

If there is evidence of disorder of the *form of thought*—to be described later—the illness is most likely to be *schizophrenia*.

In the absence of positive findings in any of these areas of the mental state, a *neurotic illness, conduct disorder or personality disorder* is likely to be diagnosed, depending on the duration and type of onset of the patient's symptomatology.

From the history and examination of the mental state, a diagnostic formulation which will form the basis of treatment will be worked out and the role of colleagues in the treatment programme decided upon. Sometimes, special investigations may be required in order to substantiate a diagnosis and usually, although not necessarily at the first visit, a physical examination will be carried out.

CLASSIFICATION

As mentioned above, a psychiatrist has had a medical training, and so has been brought up to make a clinical diagnosis and perhaps this is where the psychiatrist differs most in his method of working from professional colleagues in psychology and social work. In recent years, the so-called 'medical model' has been criticised and even some psychiatrists are beginning to doubt its validity. Yet it was because of the awareness of the causative agent in chest infections such as pneumonia or bronchitis, that penicillin was recognised as a 'wonder drug' when it first became available. One is only too well aware of the unsatisfactory state of illness-classification in psychiatry in general, and even more so in the psychiatry of the younger age groups, but it can still serve a useful function. The purpose of a classification may decide the form it should take. It may be descriptive, explanatory, prognostic or therapeutic. Drawing from the field of physical medicine, it might be considered that the ideal classification was an explanatory, or aetiological, one, but this is insufficient. For example, a classification of fractures based on a causative agent would not be helpful, whilst a description delineating the form and extent of damage round the bone is of value. Disorders can be defined, and even treated successfully, before the cause is known, as was the case with cholera and scurvy. The same agent may result in varying disease manifestations; for example the spirochaete—the organism causing syphilis—may make its major impact on the cardiovascular system or, alternatively, on the nervous system, resulting in differing clinical, pictures. To a large extent psychiatry, is at the stage of using a descriptive classification.

In adult psychiatry, there are three main diagnostic categories, neurotic illness, psychotic illness, and personality disorder. It has been said, ironically, that 'the neurotic builds castles in the air, the psychotic lives in them, and the psychiatrist collects the rent'. Neurotic illness is a disorder of the emotions, which is not accompanied by marked personality disorder, nor is the patient out of touch with reality.

In a fully developed psychotic illness, the patient loses touch with reality. In the majority of cases, in both neurotic illness and psychotic illness, a definite onset in time can be recognised before which the patient was not ill, and, if the prognosis is good, there comes a time when the patient reverts to his previous normal self, whereas in personality disorders, the difficulties have been life-long and there is no change in the life style, the behavioural pattern continuing through life, with minor modifications in the pattern relating to age.

The World Health Organisation has been developing over the years an International Classification of Disease, Injuries and Causes of Death (I.C.D.) which is used in many countries of the world. Section 5 of the I.C.D. deals with mental disorders and mental subnormality. Currently, the ninth revision is in use. In this revision, for the first time, diagnostic categories appropriate to younger-age patients have been included. These categories were based on the observations of an international working party organised by the World Health Organisation to study psychiatric disorders in childhood.

In the eighth revision of the I.C.D., the only diagnostic provision for the younger age group was Code 308; Behaviour disorder of Childhood.' It was specified that only conditions which could not be classified elsewhere should be included under this; interestingly, childhood was not defined. Similarly Code 307: 'Transient situational disturbance'—short-lived behaviour disorders of adolesence, or reactions to stressful situations were to be included: here, again, adolescence was not defined.

The ninth revision of the I.C.D. now includes categories such as:

1. Psychoses specific to childhood.
2. Disturbance of conduct.
3. Disturbance of emotion specific to childhood and adolescence.
4. Developmental disorders.
5. Hyperkinetic syndrome of childhood.

Sometimes in the younger age group, it may be important to record and classify features additional to the main clinical psychiatric syndrome, for example, if a child who is mentally handicapped, has epilepsy and a conduct-disorder which should be the main clinical psychiatric syndrome?

After much discussion, the working party on classification in child psychiatry suggested that the primary diagnosis should always reflect clinical and descriptive aspects of the psychiatric problem and that possible causative factors should be recorded on separate axes. From this arose the concept of a *multi-axial classification scheme for psychiatric disorders in childhood and adolescence*.

1. The first axis concerning the clinical psychiatric syndromes;
2. a second axis being descriptive, coding specific delay in development, *e.g.* speech, reading;
3. a third axis describing the child's level of intellectual functioning (whether regarded as contributing to the clinical psychiatric syndrome or not);
4. a fourth axis being used to record any medical condition, *e.g.*, diabetes, epilepsy, obesity, injury;
5. a fifth axis to code abnormal social conditions.

All axes refer to conditions *present* at the time of examination, and do not include *past* illnesses, psycho-social stress or developmental delay.

Definitions and detailed instruction on the use of the multi-axial classification are available now in *A Guide to a Multi-Axial Classification Scheme for Psychiatric Disorders in Childhood and Adolescence* prepared by Professor Rutter and Doctors Shaffer and Sturge, of the Institute of Psychiatry: other references give the background to the development of the multi-axial classification.

Using this guide, the following diagnostic categories will be examined in the course of the text.

1. Psychotic illness:
   a. organic psychoses
   b. childhood psychoses
   c. functional psychoses—Schizophrenia
                         The affective disorders
2. Developmental disorders, including:
   a. enopresis
   b. enuresis
   c. stuttering
   d. reading retardation
   e. hyperkinetic syndrome
   f. tics
3. Conduct disorders
4. Personality disorders
5. Emotional or neurotic disorders:
   a. anxiety states
   b. hysteria
   c. obsessional and compulsive disorders

For adolescents, it seems as though a combination of child diagnostic categories and adult diagnostic categories is required. In addition to the conventional diagnostic categories in child and adult psychiatry, some adolescents present with a recognisable symptom complex, for example, non-attendance at school, attempts at self-harm drug abuse and sexual deviation. These symptoms are sufficiently frequent to deserve examination in some detail, although, for instance, non-attendance at school can only be a symptom in a culture where education is available and expected, and therefore could never be a definite diagnostic entity. Nevertheless, there seems to be some merit in describing such syndromes.

The succeeding chapters will take up the diagnostic categories and symptom complexes of adolescence.*

EPIDEMIOLOGICAL STUDIES

The fact that disturbed adolescents are seen both at child guidance clinics and hospital psychiatric clinics may have contributed to the overall lack of information of the type of illness and the numbers presenting for treatment in this country in the younger age group. Epidemiological studies of psychiatric disturbance in adolescence are few. In this country they are confined to two surveys carried out in Scotland around the middle-60s and the results of a recent comprehensive survey carried out in the Isle of Wight are now becoming available. However, before concentrating on psychiatric problems, the situation may be put into perspective if a wider view is taken, as, by far, the majority of disturbed teenagers become involved with the law-enforcing agents such as police, Juvenile Courts, probation officers and now social workers. Although the 10–20 year-old age range makes up less than one-fifth of the total population, almost 50 per cent of those found guilty of indictable (serious) offences in England in 1971 were in this age group, and males outnumbered females eight to one. In that year, the number of males found guilty of indictable offences rose from ten years (the age of criminal responsibility), doubling at eleven and again at twelve, reaching a peak at seventeen and then slowly dropping. This picture was similar in 1970, whereas in the 1960s the peak age of male offenders was in the last year of compulsory schooling. In females, the overall figures are similar, rising from a minimum at ten to a peak at seventeen and then dwindling. The number of males found guilty of indictable offences per hundred of the population in the ten-to-twenty age group in 1971 was 3·13 and the number of females found guilty of indictable offences in this age group was 0·4 per hundred of the population at risk.†

Maladjustment is an educational term, used to describe children who show evidence of emotional instability or psychological distur-

---

* The reader new to this subject may prefer to omit the rest of this Chapter.
† Calculations based on data from *Criminal Statistics England and Wales 1971*. H.M.S.O.

bance. They may require special educational treatment in order to effect their personal, social or educational readjustment.

The Report of the Committee on Maladjusted Children (Underwood) appeared in 1955. Pilot surveys to assess the incidence of maladjustment were carried out for the committee in certain areas. In Somerset, it was found that 11·8 per cent of a random sample of 883 pupils, in Birmingham 7·7 per cent of a weighted sample of 2,264 children (6, 9 and 13 years olds), and in Berkshire 5·4 per cent of a weighted sample of 992 children, could be regarded as maladjusted. It is interesting to compare these figures with those Isle of Wight Survey discussed below.

TABLE 1
Survey of Prevalence of 'Maladjustment'

Area of Survey	Age	No. of Pupils	Prevalence of maladjustment
Somerset 1952	Random sample	883	11·8 per cent
Birmingham 1953	6, 9, 13 yrs.	2,264	7·7 per cent
Berkshire 1953	(School age)	992	5·4 per cent
Isle of Wight 1965	10–11 yrs. (total sample)	2,199	6–7 per cent
Isle of Wight 1968/9	14–15 yrs. (Total sample)	2,303	21 per cent
A London borough 1970	10 yrs.	2,281	10 per cent

Mr. Michael Britten, a psychologist with Coventry Child Guidance Clinic, presented a paper to the Royal Society of Health in May, 1970 and, using figures provided on a regular basis by the Department of Education and Science, stated that the incidence of children ascertained as maladjusted in different parts of the country varied from approximately one-twentieth of 1 per cent to one-third of 1 per cent per annum, with a wide variation between. From these figures therefore, it would appear that the majority of disturbed children are being contained within the normal educational system. Preliminary results of a survey being carried out in Newcastle-on-Tyne by Dr. Kolvin and his colleagues, would suggest perhaps that this is as it ought to be, as preliminary findings from this survey indicate that collecting grossly-disturbed children together under one roof is not necessarily the best way of helping them develop less maladaptive ways of functioning.

In what is now known as the Isle of Wight Survey, Dr. (now Professor) Michael Rutter and his colleagues used standardised questionnaires in an attempt to measure the prevalence of psychiatric disturbance on the island. These questionnaires were given to the parents and teachers of 2,199 children aged 10–11 years. On the basis of a given cut-off score, 157 children were identified for further study and 64 were finally diagnosed as having a psychiatric disorder, from the teacher's questionnaire. A similar number of children were identified from the parental questionnaire. Interestingly, only 19 were selected on both questionnaires and of these, 14 were considered to have a psychiatric disorder. This is particularly striking—how few children were picked up from both questionnaires—and this study emphasises the fact that the child who has behavioural or emotional difficulties at school may not present as a problem in the home situation, and vice versa. Out of the 2,199 children in their last year at primary school, 118 were finally diagnosed as having clinically important psychiatric disorder, representing a minimum prevalence rate of maladjustment of 5·4 per cent at this age.

A similar study was carried out by Professor Rutter and his colleagues in an inner London borough and it was found that the prevalence of psychiatric disorder there was almost double that in the Isle of Wight.

The results of a further study on the Isle of Wight, in which those children screened at 10 and 11 in the earlier 1960s were screened again by similar methods in their last year of compulsory schooling are becoming available. 2,303 children were screened in 1968–9 and again psychological disorder was diagnosed if it resulted in social impairment. A prevalence rate of emotional disturbance of 21 per cent, a significantly higher rate than that found at the 10–11 year old stage, has been found. In all studies, the important factors relating to emotional disturbance appear to be psychiatric illness in the mother, broken homes, especially where there is a history of marital discord, and one-parent families.

Independently, in the mid-1960s, the late Dr. Cecil Kidd, a psychiatrist in Edinburgh, and Dr. Caldbeck-Meenan in Belfast together carried out a study of psychiatric morbidity amongst first-year students at the two Universities, and showed that there was a marked similarity in the prevalence of psychiatric disorder—9·0 per cent of the men and 14·6 per cent of the women in Edinburgh compared with 9·1 per cent of the men and 13·5 per cent of the women in Belfast. These figures did not differ significantly from age-specific rates found among young people in the general population, when Kessell reviewed psychiatric morbidity in a London general practice.

Interestingly, the Underwood report quotes the findings of a survey by Dr. Russell Fraser, which was carried out amongst 3,000 factory workers in 1942–4. It was found that 9 per cent of the men and 13 per cent of the women had suffered from definite disabling neurotic illness during the six months prior to the survey and that a further 19 per cent of the men and 23 per cent of the women had suffered from minor degrees of neurosis during the same period. The age-range of this sample is not quoted. A study by Dr. Logan and Miss Goldberg, carried out on the physical, mental and social health of eighteen-year-old males registering for National Service in an outer borough of London in May 1949, revealed that 16 per cent of the 74 youths registering for National Service were very severely maladjusted and another 26 per cent mildly disturbed.

Epidemiology of mental illness in adolescence
Having looked at figures of estimates of disturbance in the general population, it is now appropriate to examine more closely figures relating to adolescents presenting to the psychiatric services. Two surveys give relatively detailed information. Dr. J. A. Baldwin surveyed the use made of psychiatric services in the North East of Scotland in 1965–6 and, in the United States, Dr. Beatrice Rosen examined the use made by adolescents of out-patient clinics.

Dr. Baldwin found that 783 child and adolescent patients were seen by psychiatrists in the North East of Scotland in 1965–6. The mean annual rate of referral in the region for males was 3·20 per thousand, the maximum rate of referral being 4·27 at 14 and the minimum 3·07 at 16. It is interesting to note that, for males, the maximum rate of referral at 14 was also the age at which Juvenile Court appearances were at a maximum. For females, the rate rose from 2·17 at 12 years to 8·08 per thousand at age 19. This trend confirmed the well-known observation that, proportionately, more boys than girls are seen at child guidance clinics, whereas women outnumber men in the use of adult psychiatric services. (As in other studies, mental deficiency was excluded.) When Baldwin broke his figures down into patients resident in Aberdeen (city patient) and those resident outside the urban area (country patients), lower rates of referral were seen in the country patients but, overall, the pattern was similar.

TABLE 2
Adolescent Referrals to Psychiatric Outpatient Clinics

Author	Year	Country	Age	No.	Referral rate
Rosen	1962	U.S.A.	10–20 yrs.	54,000	6·2 per thousand adolescents
Henderson et al.	1964–5	Edinburgh	14–19	230	5·6 per thousand at risk
Baldwin	1965–6	N.E. Scotland	0–20	783	Children and adolescents Male 3·20 per thousand Female 2·50 per thousand

Dr. Rosen, in the United States, says that out-patient clinics serve proportionately more persons in the 10–19 age group than in any other decade of life. She estimated that, in 1962, one quarter of the out-patients seen (194,000) were adolescents, representing 6·2 per thousand adolescents in the population. She analysed data from 788 clinics in 41 states of the U.S.A. (New York, serving 28 per cent of the adolescent population, being omitted). Of patients discharged in 1962 (a total of 54,000 patients) at 10–11 years there were 2·16 boys seen to each girl, but the number of each sex had equalised by 18 to 19 years.

Henderson and McCulloch collected data on 230 patients aged 14 to 19 years, who had at least one interview with a psychiatrist from July 1965 to June 1965, who were resident in the city of Edinburgh on the night preceding the first interview, had an I.Q. greater than 70, and had had no psychiatric consultation in the previous five years. The 230 teenagers were made up of 106 boys and 124 girls, representing an annual rate of referral to specialist services of 5·6 per thousand at risk. 51 per cent of the boys and 48 per cent of the girls had had in-patient treatment. (This seems a rather high figure, as for example, at the author's Adolescent Unit, only a quarter of the total referrals are admitted, although many referrals are specifically for in-patient treatment.)

Source of referral
Rosen found that school was the chief source of referral of both boys and girls aged between 10 to 15 years, but referrals by private physicians, teachers, family or friend were relatively frequent for young girls and for both boys and girls in their late teens. Court referrals became frequent for those aged 14–17 years, particularly boys. Rosen points out that once a child has left school, there is no institution which continues in contact or has a responsibility for him and his need to seek help, or whatever action he takes, is likely to depend on his own sense of discomfort.

In contrast, the Edinburgh survey found that half of the sample was referred by the family doctor. The teenagers so referred tended to come from the more affluent parts of the city. 10 per cent had been referred by themselves, or by relatives, and only 7 of the 230 had been referred by the Courts.

Baldwin found that over half the patients from the city and country were referred by the family doctor, but in analysing his data, it is not possible to separate referrals of younger children from those of adolescents. Referrals from Casualty Department were mainly following attempted suicide; they were few in number and none was below 12 years. Referral for a Court report was infrequent, but more common in males. This low referral from the Courts in the Edinburgh survey and Baldwin's figures may partly reflect the fact that some local authorities make independent arrangements for the psychiatric assessment of teenagers.

DIAGNOSIS
Dr. Rosen found that severe mental illness in the group accounted for fewer referrals (16 per cent) than less severe disorders (60 per cent). Under severe mental disorder, she included brain syndrome, mental deficiency and psychosis. Convulsive disorder (epilepsy)

was the most frequent brain disorder throughout the adolescent years. Less severe conditions were personality disorder, transient situational-disorders, psycho-physiological disorders and psycho-neurosis. Anxiety reaction was the most common psychoneurotic disorder, although depressive reaction amongst older girls was seen almost as frequently. Interestingly, 20 per cent of the adolescent patients were undiagnosed and 3 per cent were thought not to have a psychiatric illness. Only one-third of the patients referred were actually taken on for treatment, the remaining two-thirds receiving diagnostic assessment only. One-third of these adolescent patients discharged themselves, usually by not keeping appointments. Another third of the patients were referred to other agencies and, in fact, in only the remaining third of patients was treatment actually completed and terminated by the psychiatrist. This trend gives some indication of the frustration experienced by those working with teenage patients.

In the Aberdeen study, the use of the International Classification of Diseases was found to be unsatisfactory, so a modification of the Rutter classification referred to above was used. It was found that behaviour disorders accounted for approximately half of the referrals, the rate being higher for males than females and for city as compared with country patients. Another quarter of the referrals was on account of neurosis, the rate increasing at the age of 15, particularly in females. The rate of psychosis was low at all ages, but higher in males, tending to rise with age. 29 patients in all were diagnosed as psychotic, though the type of psychosis was not mentioned, which gives a rate of less than 0·1 per thousand.

Both Baldwin and Rosen refer to the fact that referral to psychiatric agencies may, in part, reflect the severity of a child's difficulties, but may also be an indication of the community's, (particularly the school's) degree of tolerance of such symptoms; whereas adolescent boys express their emotional conflict in sullen moods and acts of defiance, girls are more often referred because they seem listless and depressed rather than 'acting out'. Baldwin points out that the rise in the rate of referral of girls in the later teens in part reflected the increase in attempted self-harm during this age period in females. A Buckinghamshire study (Shepherd, Oppenheim and Mitchell) suggested that a control sample of children had symptoms similar to those attending a Child Guidance

Clinic, but in the patient group the symptoms were usually of a severe degree and, in addition, parental anxiety was higher and level of tolerance was lower than in the control sample.

One of the few attempts at a controlled study in relation to emotional disturbance in adolescents is that of Masterson, who reviewed 101 patients referred to a clinic, aged 12 to 18 years. 72 of these were followed up over a five-year period, and subsequently he obtained a random sample as a control group and used the same history-taking technique with it. Interestingly, the controls were found to have 1·98 symptoms as against 2·80 for patients, supporting the theory that psychiatric symptoms are not uncommon in adolescents. This was particularly so for anxiety, depression, and immaturity, which were equally common for patients and controls, but depression was more severe in the patient group and controls rarely had suicidal thoughts or attempted suicide. Masterson had anticipated that adolescents would grow out of their difficulties, but found that this was not usually the case. He also noted that the diagnostic difficulty lay, not in the choice between an adjustment-reaction of adolescence and psychiatric illness, but in determining the exact nature of the psychiatric illness. These difficulties were due to the frequent finding of more than one clinical disorder in the presenting picture and the unclear definition of diagnostic categories; resolution of the diagnostic dilemma occurred only with the passage of time.

This review of some of the studies available relating to the nature and size of the problems of adolescence presenting to the psychiatrist indicates the need for further studies and also underlines the frustrations likely to be encountered by those attempting to obtain co-operation from this age group.

REFERENCES AND FURTHER READING

Baldwin, J. A. 'Psychiatric Illness from Birth to Maturity; An Epidemiological Study. Acta Psychiatric. Scandinavica, 1968, *44*, 313.

Britten, M. *The Epidemiology of Maladjustment.* Lecture read May, 1970. Royal Society of Health.

Graham. P. 'Psychiatric Disorders in the Young Adolescent: A follow-up study.' Proc. Roy. Soc. Med., 1973, *6*, 1226.

Henderson, A. S., McCulloch, J. W. and Phillip, A. E. 'Survey of Mental Illness in Adolescents.' British Medical Journal, 1967, *1*, 83.

H.M.S.O. *Report of the Committee on Maladjusted Children*—Ministry of Education, 1955. (Underwood Report).

Kidd, C. B. 'Comparative Study of Psychiatric Morbidity Amongst Students at Two Different Universities. Brit. J. Psych. 1966, *122*, 57.

Kolvin, I. *Lecture at Conference of the Association Child Psychology and Psychiatry*, London 1974.

Logan, R. S. L. 'Rising 18 in a London Suburb.' Brit. J. Sociol., 1953, *4*, 323.

Masterson, J. F. *Psychiatric Dilemma of Adolescence.* Little, Brown & Co. 1967.

*Rosen, B. M., Bahn, A. K., Shellow, R. and Bower, E. M. 'Adolescent Patients served in Out-patient Psychiatric Clinics.' American Journal of Public Health, 1965, *55*, 1563.

*Rutter, M. 'Classification and Categorisation in Child Psychiatry.' Journal of Child Psychology and Psychiatry, 1965, 671.

Rutter, M. 'Why are London Children so Disturbed?' Proc. Roy. Soc. Med., 1973, *66*, 1221.

Rutter, M., Lebovici, S., Eisenberg, L., Sneznevskij, A. D., Sadoun, R., Brooke, E. and Tsung-Yi Lin. 'A Triaxial Classification of Mental Disorders in Childhood—An International Study.' Journal of Child Psychology and Psychiatry, 1969, *10*, 41.

Rutter, M., Tizard, J. and Whitmore, K. *Educational, Health and Behaviour.* Longman, 1970.

*Rutter, M., Shaffer, D. and Sturge, C. (prepared by). *A Guide to a Multi-axial Classification Scheme for Psychiatric Disorders in Childhood and Adolescence.* Institute of Psychiatry, 1975.

Shepherd, M., Cooper, N., Brown, A. C. and Kalten, S. W. *Psychiatric Illness in General Practice.* Oxford University Press, 1966.

Shepherd, M., Oppenheim, A. W. and Mitchell, S. 'Childhood Behaviour Disorders and Child Guidance Clinic: an Epidemiological Study.' J. Psychol and Psychiat., 1966, *7*, 39.

West, D. J. *The Young Offender.* Penguin Books, 1967.

* *Recommended selected reading*

4 The organic psychoses in adolescence including the childhood psychoses

The word 'psychosis' is derived from the Greek *psyche* meaning 'mind' and *osis* meaning a 'state' or 'condition' and has come to imply a disorder of the mind. The term is said to have been first employed by Von Feuchtersleben in 1854 although it did not come into general use until this century, the word 'insanity' being used instead. With the passage of time, the word psychosis has acquired a relatively specific meaning. Psychotic illnesses are the most serious of mental illnesses, in the sense that patients suffering from these conditions are out of touch with reality, their whole personality is involved, and, whilst suffering from the illness, there is an impairment of social adjustment. Traditionally, the psychotic illnesses are divided into two groups:

1. The organic psychoses: those where there are demonstrable underlying physical causes.
2. The functional psychoses those where no specific physical cause has been shown.

The functional psychoses are further divided into the schizophrenias and the affective psychoses (disturbance of mood).

53

THE ORGANIC PSYCHOSES
The organic psychoses may be:

a. Acute

b. Chronic

Acute organic psychoses

Before antibiotics became available, childhood illnesses were frequently associated with delirium, a complication rarely seen today. Similarly, after childbirth, many women might become delirious as a result of a breast abcess or infection of the womb, but with better methods of prevention and control of infection, the pattern of mental illness following delivery has altered. Acute organic psychoses are rare in adolescence, but may occasionally be seen in relation to an obscure infection, systemic upset or drug abuse.

Clinical picture

An acute organic psychosis is a condition in which the patient is less aware of his surroundings than normal and it may vary from a state of reduced wakefulness, right up to unconsciousness and coma. In such a state, the patient often shows an impairment of *orientation*, in that he may be unaware of the time of day, the date, or which day of the week it is; he may not recognise where he is and may misidentify people in his immediate environment, for example, confusing the hospital with prison, mistaking the nursing staff for warders, or for teachers in a school; it may be difficult to gain the patient's attention for any length of time and this *impairment of attention* is commonly seen in organic mental states. The patient may manifest a symptom known as *perseversation*, that is, a tendency to repeat things such as words or actions unnecessarily. The patient may have a disturbance of *perception* commonly manifested by *illusions and hallucinations*.

Illusions are the misinterpretation of perceptions in the presence of an environmental stimulus; for example, a piece of paper may be misinterpreted as a snake. Hallucinations are disturbances of perception in the absence of any external stimulus. Hallucinations may involve sight, when they are known as visual hallucinations, hearing—auditory hallucinations, smell—olfactory hallucinations or touch—tactile hallucinations. Visual hallucinations are those most commonly seen in association with organic mental states. Hallucinations may be so frightening that the patient is reduced to a state of terror by them.

Diagnosis
By definition, an organic mental state is associated with underlying physical factors. There may be actual brain pathology, or a metabolic or biochemical disturbance, which disrupts brain function and gives rise to the characteristics and symptoms described in the clinical picture. If an organic mental state is suspected, a search for the underlying cause is essential. The causes include:

a. Infections
b. Exogenous intoxication, for example, drugs and poisons
c. Metabolic upset (endogenous intoxication) for example, the uraemia of kidney failure
d. Cerebral causes

Until recently, infections were the commonest cause of acute organic syndromes in adolescence, but nowadays drug-misuse is seen more commonly, so that when a patient presents with the diagnosis of an organic mental state, the question of an overdose of drugs must be considered. An overdose of some of the psychotropic drugs (*i.e.*, capable of modifying mental activity), such as anti-depressants, may give rise to unusual symptoms without marked impairment of consciousness and, if drug misuse is not suspected, diagnostic difficulties can arise. The question of lead intoxication or other industrial chemicals must also be kept in mind, particularly in the young wage-earner who may ignore rudimentary safety precautions. Metabolic disorders giving rise to unconsciousness are usually fairly readily recognised but, occasionally, drug-takers may neglect their diet and secondary malnutrition with vitamin deficiency may contribute to an abnormal mental state. Cerebral causes include mental disorder associated with a head injury, with an infection such as meningitis or encephalitis, and with space-occupying lesions (tumours). Cerebral haemorrhage and thrombosis are rare in adolescence, but occasionally occur. Confusional states may also be associated with epilepsy.

Treatment
Even if the cause giving rise to the organic mental state has been identified, admission to hospital will almost always be necessary. The main treatment is that of the underlying illness, but this will not be discussed further here. The management of the confusional episode, however, is also important. While the patient is mentally disturbed, he should be nursed in a well-lighted room, the light being kept on throught the night. He should not be left alone and restraint, in particular bed-rails, should be avoided. The purpose of these precautions is to prevent the patient misidentifying objects in his environment and generally to reduce the degree of confusion. Acute symptoms will be controlled by drugs such as one of the phenothiazine group, for example chlorpromazine, or one of the butyrophenones such as haloperidol (*see* Chapter 18). Good basic nursing skills are important, including supervision of adequate fluid intake and attention to bladder and bowels, skin care, and mouth and overall hygiene.

Prognosis
The outlook in the acute organic mental state is usually good in relation to the acute mental symptoms, but the overall prognosis obviously depends on the underlying cause and, in some instances, the patient may be left with a residual chronic organic psychosis.

Chronic organic psychoses
A chronic organic mental state may arise *de novo*, or may be the end result of an acute organic mental state. The most commonly seen chronic organic mental state is dementia, which usually occurs in the 'second childhood' associated with old age, rather than with adolescence but, sadly, some teenagers who suffer from illnesses such as encephalitis, the end-result of a head injury, complications arising from diabetic coma, epilepsy or cerebral haemorrhage, may remain permanently brain-damaged.
Clinical features The whole picture is less dramatic than that of the acute organic mental state and there may either be a history of a preceding acute episode, or else the onset of the symptoms is more insidious. In general, the main area of disturbance is that of cognitive function. The patient may be disorientated for time, place and person and he may suffer from a disorder of attention and be

distractible. Often, one obtains a history of a marked change in personality and from being a placid, cheerful individual, he may become irritable and show marked lack of inhibition in his speech and behaviour. The inability to sustain attention, and the disinhibition, may make it difficult for the individual to continue with academic learning. Occasionally, disturbance may be so marked that it becomes impossible for the youngster to remain in the community and long-term care in hospital may be necessary. The less handicapped are potentially able to remain at home, but their families must have adequate support, both physical and emotional.

The effect on his developing brothers and sisters of having a handicapped youngster in the home must also be taken into consideration. It may be important, for example, to arrange re-admission of the youngster with long-term handicaps for holidays, so that families may arrange for their own holiday, though equally, it is not possible to overburden hospitals in the summer months when the hospital staff themselves are often very stretched. Apart from some of the better mental subnormality hospitals, facilities for children with chronic organic mental states are poorly developed. Those of normal intelligence are small in number, but the problem that they present is quite out of proportion to their numbers in the community. In many instances they are best helped by those with expertise in mental subnormality (see Chapter 16).

In adolescence, many with psychiatric handicaps are ostracised by their contemporaries and most will be seriously distressed by this rejection. As they become more adult, and their contemporaries also age, there may be an improvement in mutual tolerance. These handicapped children often require a particularly sheltered environment in the fields of education and employment. They may have difficulty in re-learning socially acceptable behaviour and often the reasonably structured-regime, such as is used in helping those with a mental handicap, is valuable. It is important to spell things out to them in terms of black and white, as it may be difficult for such patients to work out decisions and plans of action for themselves.

The use of psychotropic drugs can control particular aspects of behaviour and may be useful in some instances (see Chapter 18).

*   *   *

Before moving on to consider schizophrenia and the affective ill-nesses, we come to a small diagnostic no-man's land. A few children develop psychotic illnesses which were traditionally thought to be of psychological origin. Nowadays, there is in-creasing evidence that organic factors play an important part in the causation of at least some of them, so it is perhaps better to men-tion them briefly at this point.

Psychotic illness in childhood
The psychoses in childhood are divided into three main groups depending on the age at onset:

1. Infantile autism.
2. Psychoses of early childhood.
3. Psychoses of late childhood.

Infantile autism
This was first described by Kanner in 1943. The onset of this illness occurs within the first two to three years of life and is characterised by autism (an aloofness, a failure to form human relationships, with marked social withdrawal), impaired speech development, and ritualistic behaviour with a reluctance to accept change. Boys are more commonly affected than girls and there is evidence of some association with higher social groups. The majority of children with infantile autism will have been diagnosed in early childhood and ap-propriate arrangements for their education should have been made long before adolescence. However, there is a tendency for some of these children to develop epilepsy in adolescence and they may pre-sent to the psychiatrist on this account. Children with infantile autism have some capacity to improve slowly and there is now some evidence that they may only begin to learn efficiently in adolescence if they can be kept in an educational environment. On the whole, however, the patient is more likely to come in contact with a specialist in mental subnormality and then at a later stage, the general psychiatrist.

Childhood psychoses
These have their onset in middle childhood. Children presenting with this type of illness have a history of normal development until

the age of three to five years, following which there is a pattern of regression. It seems that the majority of children developing a psychotic illness between the ages of three and eight show evidence of degenerative disease, although on clinical examination there may be no abnormalities detected in the nervous system. These children appear to have a particularly poor prognosis and become long-stay patients in mental subnormality hospitals, or, occasionally, adult psychiatric wards. On balance it would seem that mental subnormality hospitals have more to offer in management and in practical terms these childhood psychoses are probably best considered with the chronic organic mental states described earlier.

Late-onset psychoses in childhood
Here the psychotic illness develops after the age of eight and tends to be similar in form to adult schizophrenia which will be described below. In this group, possible organic causes are very much less certain.

REFERENCES AND FURTHER READING

Curran, D., Partridge, M., Storey, P. Chapter 6, 'Organic Mental states' in *Psychological Medicine, An Introduction to Psychiatry*. Churchill Livingstone, 7th Edtn., 1972.

Rutter, M. (ed.). *Infantile Autism: Concepts, Characteristics and Treatment*. Churchill Livingstone, 1971.

Rutter, M. 'Psychotic Disorders in Early Childhood', Chapter 10 in *Recent Developments Schizophrenia'*—A Symposium. Ed. Coppen A. and Walk, A. Published for Royal Medico-Psychological Association by Headley Brothers Limited, 1967.

Wing, L. (Ed.). *Early Childhood Autism*. Pergamon Press, 2nd ed. 1975.

Wing, L. 'Syndome of Early Childhood Autism' in 'Contempory Psychiatry'—selected Reviews from Brit. J. Psychiatry. Ed. Silverstone, T. and Barraclough, B. Brit. J. Psych., Special Publication No. 9. Headley Brothers Ltd., 1975.

5 Schizophrenia

The word 'schizophrenia' is derived from the Greek and means 'split mind'. It was introduced to replace an older name for this illness: 'Dementia praecox' or the 'insanity of youth', as opposed to senile dementia, which is the insanity of old age. As psychiatrists became aware that the illness now called schizophrenia differed from dementia, they realised that there was no impairment of consciousness or memory as is seen with organic mental states, but that there were often disorders of thinking and of feeling, with disorganisation of the patient's personality. So the term schizophrenia became preferred to the misleading 'precocious dementia'. The illness is characterised by a disorder of thinking, feeling and motor-activity, with disorganisation of the personality.

CLINICAL PICTURE

The onset of schizophrenic illness may be gradual or acute. The patient with an insidious onset progressively withdraws into himself and appears increasingly apathetic. As a result of this, he has less contact with friends and tends to spend more and more time in his own world, which may be dominated by fantasies and/or delusions. Many young schizophrenics become preoccupied with philosophical ideas, so that at times it may be difficult to say whether these are a normal adolescent preoccupation, or whether they may be the first sign of a serious psychotic illness. Those who know the patient well may recognise a change in his personality, bordering on oddity or eccentricity. The patient himself may be perplexed by the change which he notices in himself during the early stages of the illness and it is only in the full-blown illness that his insight may be lost. A feeling of perplexity is, in fact, the most marked mood-change in the young schizophrenic. At times he may appear depressed, but on closer observation it usually emerges that apathy describes the mood change better than dejection.

When the onset is more acute, the patient may suddenly develop florid symptoms and complain that he is being spied on, or that his food is being poisoned, or he may express other unusual ideas. The particularly-disturbed schizophrenic expressing such anxieties may act on them and it is with this type of presentation that violence, although rare, may occur. The schizophrenic patient often feels that other people are talking about him or persecuting him and although there is no basis for this in reality, he may attack the person whom he regards as his persecutor. Occasionally, in an acutely disturbed state, the patient may kill himself rather than those with whom he is angry.

At the beginning of a schizophrenic illness, doctors have learnt to look for particular symptoms which may be categorised as:

1. Disorders of thinking.
2. Disorders of emotion.
3. Disorders of will and volition.
4. Disorders of motor activity.
5. Hallucinations.

Disorders of thinking
These may result in an alteration in the speed or the coherence of thinking, an alteration of the form of thinking, or there may be disorder of the thought-content. For example, thoughts may come quickly or slowly; normally, we have learnt to express our thoughts in terms which others can follow without difficulty and in logical sequence, but in some forms of mental illness, this process of logical thinking is disrupted and the patient may begin expressing

his thoughts on one theme and then suddenly introduce a new and unconnected idea. Linked with this is a phenomenon in which thinking just appears to stop for a short time and this is termed 'thought blocking' and is characteristic of schizophrenia, though it may also occur to a lesser extent in other situations, for example, in a very anxious person.

There may be a marked loosening in the association of ideas and, as well as this, a person who could formerly think in abstract terms may resort to thinking in concrete terms (Chapter 2). Some patients with schizophrenia may experience *alienation* of thought, in the sense that their thinking becomes foreign to them. They may feel that they are being deprived of their thoughts; that thoughts are being inserted into their minds; or, alternatively, that their thoughts are being broadcast. This particular form of thought-disorder is very characteristic of schizophrenia.

A delusion is a false belief which does not respond to reason and is foreign to the patient's culture. The disorder of thought content in many schizophrenics takes the form of delusional beliefs, although delusions themselves may occur in other illnesses, so that the presence of such ideas is not exclusively diagnostic of schizophrenia. Patients may express the conviction that their thoughts are being affected from outside, perhaps by telepathy or electronic rays. Schizophrenics may also express delusions of persecution. Although, by definition, delusions are foreign to the patient's in- dividual culture, they must also be related to his life's experience, so that, for example, several centuries ago it would not have been possible for patients to experience delusions related to electronics or atomic energy. Then they were more likely to have delusions related to religious beliefs.

Delusions may take several forms; they may be *persecutory* in which the patient complains of someone deliberately plotting to harm him; *grandiose*, in which the patient believes he has got some special powers, such as that he is a particularly important person, or of superior intelligence; *hypochondriacal*, in which he becomes preoccupied with bodily function, and may express such bizarre ideas as that his insides have dropped out; *nihilistic* in which the patient may believe that he has actually died; *erotic* delusions, when a patient may believe that someone of the opposite sex has a particular interest in him.

Disorders of emotion

Mood disturbances may occur in several forms, and patients may be dispirited, high spirited or anxious. These are normal variations which we all experience, but when a person is dejected over a long period of time, we refer to this as depression and pathologically-sustained high-spiritedness we describe as a state of elation. These and anxiety are mood-changes which may predominate in schizophrenia, but in view of the fact that there is also evidence of thought-disorder, the diagnosis is one of schizophrenia rather than of affective psychosis (*see* later). There is some evidence that marked emotional disturbance, in association with thought disorder in schizophrenia, is an important prognostic factor; if the mood disturbance is marked, the outlook tends to be better. Apart from these particular mood changes, the schizophrenic may exhibit other features, such as lack of emotion or warmth, or inappropriateness of mood. A shallowness of affect with loss of finer feelings may be noted. Relatives may become aware of these changes early in the illness, but the patient's own capacity for insight varies very much from individual to individual.

Disturbances of volition (initiative)

Many schizophrenics develop lack of initiative and loss of spontaneity, associated with a lack of energy, loss of drive and indecisiveness. These may be early symptoms in the illness. As a result of these difficulties, the patient's hygiene may deteriorate and he loses interest in his personal appearance. The outcome of this particular group of symptoms is often that where a patient has attended work regularly he may now have difficulty in getting up in the morning and be unable to undertake the work even if he gets there. Then, he may eventually lose his job or require to transfer to a less demanding task. Where these features become extremely marked, a condition of *stupor* occasionally arises, in which there is absence of speech and movement although the patient is conscious.

Disorders of motor activity

The opposite of stupor may be seen in patients with over-activity, which may even progress to a state of pathological excitement. This is particularly seen in catatonic schizophrenia (*see* below). Sometimes these outbursts of activity are a response to an hallucinatory voice. Schizophrenic patients may show repetitive meaningless movements such as rocking backwards and forwards, rubbing themselves or objects, or they may adopt unusual stances which they can maintain for a long time, but such florid disturbances of external behaviour can now usually be quickly helped with treatment and have become much less common.

Hallucinations
These are abnormal sensory perceptions as, for example, when a patient may claim that an abnormal odour is invading the atmosphere, when no unusual smell is noticed by others present. Perhaps the commonest form of hallucinations known to the general public are *visual* hallucinations discussed in the previous chapter. Tactile hallucinations may occur when a patient claims to have been touched or have sensations like insects crawling over him. However, the commonest form of hallucination in schizophrenia is the *auditory* hallucination, in which a patient may hear voices, which take the form of a statement, or may present as a running commentary on his behaviour. Sometimes he may hear his own thoughts spoken aloud. The voices which the patient hears tend to be objectionable and they may be threatening or abusive; occasionally they may terrify the patient; if the voices give orders, the patient may feel obliged to carry these out. Sometimes a patient hears his own thoughts almost before he thinks them, as if they were dictated to him, or he may feel that they are being inserted into his mind. On occasions, he may hear his thoughts immediately afterwards like an 'echo'. Hallucinatory voices are experienced as coming from outside the patient's head in contradistinction to pseudo-hallucinations, which are experienced inside the head.

DIAGNOSIS

The diagnosis of schizophrenia is based on the observation of a combination of those symptoms just described, although few of them are exclusive to schizophrenia. Most of them may be encountered in other diseases and even in normal people, particularly at times of stress; many people experience 'voices' as they are falling off to sleep, which are known as hypnagogic hallucinations and are not regarded as abnormal.

According to the combination of symptoms, four different types of schizophrenia are usually recognised. These are:

1. Hebephrenic schizophrenia (from the Greek *hebe*, meaning youth): The patient acts in a silly, childish fashion. This type of schizophrenia is dominated by thought disorder, associated with emotional disturbance and lack of initiative. The onset is usually insidious, it rarely occurs before puberty but the incidence markedly increases between puberty and early adult life.

2. Simple schizophrenia: This is perhaps the most difficult type of schizophrenia to diagnose, as the diagnosis is based on negative rather than positive symptoms.

The most helpful feature in making the diagnosis is a clear-cut account from the relatives of a marked change in the patient's personality. For example, from being a considerate youth with an interest in the usual teenage activities, he becomes withdrawn, showing a marked lack of consideration for other people.

3. Catatonic schizophrenia: In this group, motor-symptoms predominate. This type of schizophrenia is more likely to develop after the age of twenty and appears to be seen less commonly now than some decades ago. The onset is frequently acute, presentation being either with stupor or a state of excitement. The patient often acts impulsively and may be a danger to himself or to others.

4. Paranoid schizophrenia: The onset of this type of schizophrenia is usually in adult life. Although paranoid ideas (particularly persecutory delusions) may appear in other types of schizophrenia, it is the delusional aspect which predominates in this group. In contradistinction to other types of schizophrenia, the personality is often quite well preserved in paranoid schizophrenia.

FACTORS CONTRIBUTING TO SCHIZOPHRENIA

It is likely that, ultimately, it will be found that the cause of schizophrenia is metabolic or biochemical, but as yet no definite cause is known. The fact that it is rare before puberty could be interpreted as suggestive of a relationship with the biochemical changes at this time of life. Genetic factors have been studied and data available from twin studies and from families in which there appears to be an excessive tendency for schizophrenia to occur, support the view that there is an hereditary predisposition to schizophrenia, though it is unlikely to be a single gene. It may be that, even if an individual carries the gene, it is still necessary for other factors to appear before he actually develops schizophrenia.

It has long been recognised that many schizophrenics have shown rather unusual personalities before the illness developed. Before the appearance of the illness about half of the patients will have noticed to be shy and rather withdrawn individuals, tending to be over-sensitive and somewhat suspicious. Whilst undoubtedly many of those who develop schizophrenia may have such so-called schizoid personalities, little work has been done to follow up individuals with schizoid personalities to see how many of them, and under what circumstances, develop schizophrenia. It has been noted that schizophrenia is unusual in people of so called pyknic build (people of this build tend to appear stocky with relatively short neck and limbs and rather large trunks). Many of these people tend to be overweight (the John Bull type). On the other hand, the asthenic (that is the tall, thin individual with poor muscle development and a tendency to stoop) appears to be more liable than average to develop schizophrenia.

There is a school of thought in which it is considered that the environment may be important in making genetic predispositions manifest, but although many studies of parental attitudes and the degree of previous socialisation have been carried out, the results are inconclusive.

TREATMENT AND MANAGEMENT

In the opinion of the author, schizophrenia is such a serious illness that it is vital that the correct diagnosis be made at the outset. Preferably, this should be done in a hospital inpatient setting, as the implications of the diagnosis are far-reaching and a period of observation is usually needed to confirm it. If a teenager is acutely disturbed at the outset of the illness, he may best be nursed on an adult ward and later be introduced into a ward where the other patients are of his own age. There is a serious likelihood that he will be actively rejected by his age peers if he is admitted to an adolescent ward at the outset, as teenagers are very concerned about the stigma of madness and the admission of an acutely hallucinated youngster increases their anxiety to an intolerable level.

Until the cause is known, there will be no actual cure for schizophrenia, but with modern methods the disease can often be brought under control sufficiently for patients to lead a fairly active life in the community, whereas in the first half of this century, many schizophrenics were condemned to prolonged sojourn in psychiatric institutions.

First of all, the acute symptoms are brought under control with medication. The drugs most commonly used are those belonging to the phenothiazine group and the butyrophenones. Details of these are given in Chapter 18. As the patient's concentration improves and it is possible to make contact with him, he is encouraged to take part in a ward-based activity programme. This includes occupational therapy, where the patient joins with others in a group occupation. He should be encouraged to express his own preferences and in the early stages of the illness, he ought to be stimulated by being offered a variety of activities. (For the young schizophrenic, industrial therapy, with its tendency towards repetitive production-line work, should not be used in the acute stages of the illness). The patient should also be encouraged to take part in general social activities such as debates, quizzes and dancing. It may well be that his thinking will be too disturbed for him to concentrate and contribute actively to these activities, but he may subsequently admit that he gained from inclusion in them because they 'kept him in touch'. Games and physical recreation may also be valuable at this stage, particularly if the patient has a previous interest in athletic pursuits. It is here that a detailed knowledge of the patient's previous interests and personality is particularly valuable in helping to stimulate him and reintegrate him, first in the ward situation and then outside in the larger community. The aim of treatment is to persuade the patient to live in the real world, rather than the world which has been created by his illness, thus a treatment such as psychoanalysis is contra-indicated, as patients in analysis are encouraged to be introspective and this is detrimental to a schizophrenic.

Many patients will need help with hygiene and their personal appearance. It is important that good habits are established during the period in hospital and that the patients are encouraged to develop a healthy routine. For example, it is quite wrong to let women go around with stockings slipping down to their ankles, as this will make them conspicuous on their return to the community and may contribute to ostracisation and subsequent break-down.

As the acute symptoms come under control, the patient will be allowed out of hospital for periods of leave, the length of time gradually increasing. Particularly for the young schizophrenic, it is important that the family are aware of the difficulties relating to the illness and in what aspects special allowances should be made. It is important, however, that when at home on brief leave, the patient should not be treated as a guest but should be expected to help with washing dishes, laying the table and other household chores as far as his mental state permits. With younger adolescents, parents may be so distressed by the illness that they become over-indulgent, giving large amounts of money and showering them with presents. Eventually they will have cause to regret this, as schizophrenic teenagers can be just as manipulative and demanding as their healthier brethren. In the acute stages of the illness visitors, particularly people from outside the family, should be restricted in numbers but once this phase is over, contact with friends who will take the adolescent to discotheques, youth clubs, badminton clubs, etc., should be encouraged.

Circumstances indicate at what stage the patient should gradually be weaned back into the community; if his home is near enough to the hospital it may be the most obvious step for him to have bed and breakfast at home, returning to hospital as a day patient. Alternatively, if the hospital is some distance from his home, he may find a job halfway between home and hospital, so that he can become established at work before returning home. Obviously local factors, such as availability of employment, will have to be taken into account. Occasionally, employment in a sheltered workshop may be a necessary intermediate step.

There is some evidence to suggest that exacerbation of the schizophrenic illness may be brought about by highly-charged emotional situations, such as may occur in a closely knit family. If a family is in a state of upheaval (sometimes as a result of the illness) it may be advisable for a schizophrenic patient to live in a hostel or lodgings, rather than return home. It is important that lodgings are known to hospital staff, as occasionally unscrupulous people will exploit schizophrenics; accommodation, diet and heating may be inadequate, so that diseases associated with unsavoury conditions, such as scurvy or scabies may occur. Unfortunately, few landlords or landladies are willing or able to provide the supervision in terms of hygiene and appearance which many schizophrenics require. This may become less important as hospitals are becoming more aware of such problems and patients are being taught to care for themselves before being discharged from hospital, whereas in the past the tendency was for them to have everything done for them in hospital, so that any small degree of initiative they might have had was stifled.

Frequently, schizophrenia is a recurring illness. The outlook for a first attack is good, especially where the onset has been acute, in those of pyknic build, and where there was a sound previous personality. In many instances, following a first attack, the patient will return to his previous level of functioning and may be able to resume his place in the community. Should he have a recurrence, it may be found that, when the acute symptoms subside, the patient will have lost some of his initiative. Just as in chest disease, the patient with a first attack of bronchitis may be left with a perfectly healthy chest, with recurring attacks he may have a tendency to develop a persistent cough and, eventually, secondary effects on his heart, so with the schizophrenic patient: if he is subject to repeated attacks, he becomes less able to make use of his intelligence and personality. In particular, he is likely to show a lack of initiative and spontaneity. Where a patient is handicapped to this extent, sheltered workshop or industrial therapy within the hospital setting may be beneficial. It is recognised that many schizophrenic patients are in danger of having a syndrome of *institutionalisation* grafted on to their schizophrenia; it is also true that patients with schizophrenia are particularly easy to institutionalise. The patient who has been in a general hospital for many years, on account of a physical handicap, will have much less difficulty in reintegrating into the community than a schizophrenic patient.

As with the mentally handicapped (*see* Chapter 16), when the majority of schizophrenic patients lived in single-sex wards in hospital, the question of marriage and conception did not arise, but now, with the patients returning to live in the community, questions such as this pose quite a problem. With the currently earlier age of marriage, it may be that some patients will have married before the onset of the illness. Fortunately, there is evidence to suggest that fertility in schizophrenia is low, but in some instances children will have been born before the schizophrenic illness develops. Where a patient has once had a schizophrenic illness, the possibility of a recurrence always exists and a future spouse should be aware of the risks. The majority of family doctors and psychiatrists who know that a patient is contemplating matrimony, will ask permission to have a frank discussion with the patient's fiancé, so that he or she may be aware of the responsibility being taken on. For the female schizophrenic, there is a distinct possibility that, should she become pregnant, she may have a further schizophrenic episode following delivery of the child. The risk of this is thought by many to be sufficiently high to justify termination of the pregnancy, but many schizophrenics may show no deterioration in their mental state in relation to pregnancy, so that the effect of one childbirth may be acceptable.

In view of the genetic aspects of schizophrenia, prospective parents may be anxious about the likelihood of offspring being predisposed to schizophrenia. There is no doubt that a schizophrenic parent presents a serious risk to the child, thought to be of the order of 12 per cent. On account of possible deterioration in a schizophrenic mother's health, we must always consider the likely effects on her child, so contraception and family planning ought to be freely available to all schizophrenic patients.

Schizophrenic parents may also create other problems for offspring. Professor Michael Rutter in his monograph *Children of Sick Parents* showed that both physically and psychiatrically ill parents were likely to have children with more emotional problems than children of healthy parents. This is particularly the case with the child of a psychiatrically-ill parent who has been involved in the symptoms of the parental illness. At times, it may seem that by returning schizophrenic parents to the community we are almost condemning their offspring to institutionalisation, since quite a number of their children may have to be taken into care or be sent to boarding school on account of emotional problems.

REFERENCES AND FURTHER READING

Anderson, E. W. and Trethowan, W. H. Chapter 9 'Schizophrenia' in *Psychiatry*. Ballière Tindall, 3rd. Edtn., 1973.

Coppen, A. and Walk, A. *Recent Developments in Schizophrenia* (A Symposium). Publ. For Royal Medic. Psychological Assoc. by Headley Brothers Ltd., 1967.

Hamilton, M. (Ed.), Fish's *Clinical Psychopathology*. John Wright and Sons Ltd., 1974.

Rutter, M. *Children of Sick Parents: An Environmental and Psychiatric Study*. Institute of Psychiatry. Maudsley Monograph No. 16. Oxford University Press, 1966.

Sim, M. Chapter 13 'Schizophrenia' in *A Guide to Psychiatry*. Churchill Livingstone, 3rd Ed., 1974.

Slater, E. and Roth, M. Chapter 5 'Schizophrenia' in *Clinical Psychiatry*. Ballière, Tindall and Cassell, 3rd Edtn., 1969.

6 Affective illness

The *Glossary of Mental Disorders* defines affective psychoses as 'Disorders characterised by morbid changes of mood in the form of depression or excitement. They usually appear unprovoked, but may occasionally follow some form of stress. They have a tendency to recur and are self-limiting, *i.e.,* reversion to the normal nearly always occurs in time and may be hastened with treatment.' Two main types of this illness are seen in adolescence:

1. The manic type.
2. The depressive type.

THE MANIC TYPE

Definition
'This is characterised by marked mood change in the direction of elation or excitement, out of keeping with the patient's circumstances' (*Glossary of Mental Disorders*).

Clinical features
The patient shows disturbance of mood, disturbance of movement and disturbance of thinking. This mood may range from an infectious gaiety to marked elation and it influences behaviour to such

72

an extent that the patient feels all-powerful, will often brook no interference, and becomes uninhibited in his behaviour. He is usually
over-active, rushing around purposelessly. Superficially, he appears
to have a lot of initiative, but he does not follow his ideas through
and his interest in projects is not sustained. His thoughts crowd in on
one another, and this pressure of thought may be shown by the fact
that the patient never stops talking and may even become hoarse.
Characteristically, he jumps from one topic to another, the
sequence of his conversation being dictated by chance association
rather than by logic. He may express ideas about his supreme intellectual capacity or his wealth, or exhibit other grandiose ideas.

Many manic patients talk about their love affairs and many
become entangled in an erotic situation. As the depressed patient
may actually commit suicide, so it is sometimes said that the manic
patient is liable to commit social suicide; for example, by making
an exhibition of himself in a public place, on account of his uninhibited speech and behaviour, or by spending large sums of
money which he believes he possesses on account of his grandiose
state. It may prove difficult for others to restrain the individual, so
that a woman may sometimes run up big dress bills, or a man may
buy cars or houses, or undertake major business deals which he
does not have the expertise or financial backing to carry through (a
feature of a manic illness which makes it important to recognise at
an early stage). If in-patient treatment is required, it may be
necessary to admit the patient to hospital under a Section of the
Mental Health Act, as he is unlikely to recognise that he is ill, and
even if he agrees to come into hospital, he may decide to discharge
himself after a very brief stay. If he is under treatment at this time,
it may be difficult to find sufficient evidence to detain him in
hospital and yet, once he is out of hospital, he is likely to stop
taking his medicines and perhaps recreate the problems which
brought about his admission in the first instance, again exhibiting
unhibited behaviour and talking indiscreetly.

Management
Drugs are the main method of treatment in mania; again, as the
cause has not yet been established, treatment is essentially symptomatic (*see* below).

One of the phenothiazines such as chlorpromazine or a

butyrophenone such as haloperidol will be used to control the condition in the first instance. If the situation does not improve and come under control rapidly, E.C.T. (electro-convulsive therapy) may be given, but this is now used less frequently in the treatment of mania than in the past. Recently, the use of lithium in order to prevent further attacks has been applied and can be very effective. For details of drug treatment the reader is referred to Chapter 18.

It is always difficult to reason with manic patients, as they do not appreciate that they are ill. It may be embarrassing and harmful for the patient and relatives should the patient indulge in an orgy of letter-writing or make frequent telephone calls, both of which activities may be indiscreetly carried out. Many doctors explain to patients that it is important that they have a rest and if they write letters the recipient is bound to reply. So, even if they write letters to relieve their own feelings, it is important that they should not be posted if the patient is agreeable. By doing this, an attempt can be made to reduce some of the social repercussions that are likely to arise if the patient is allowed to continue acting in an uninhibited way.

In adults, sleep disturbance is usually a prominent feature of a manic phase of illness, but in adolescents this symptom is often less obvious. In some adolescents, the uninhibited conversation and behaviour may be attributed to cheekiness when the attack is mild, or in the initial stages of a more serious episode, and so the diagnosis may be overlooked.

THE DEPRESSIVE TYPE

Definition
'In depression the mood is one of dejection which is out of keeping with the circumstances of the patient.'

Clinical description
A feeling of dejection may arise because of unpleasant circumstances, for example learning that an examination has been failed, or following an argument with a boy-friend. The reason for the sad feeling is obvious to everyone, including the patient. Usually, such a feeling is not unduly prolonged, although occasionally it may persist. Some people, on account of their personalities, create

situations which may make them unpopular and they may experience a degree of misery on account of this, but again, they may be able to understand the reason for their feelings and, if they wish, may be able to take steps to improve the situation. However, in the more serious depressive illness described below, the reason for the depression may not be obvious and, as will be discussed later, may be related to biochemical changes in the brain.

The degree of depression arising in these circumstances may be so mild that the individuals themselves would hardly dignify it by the word 'depression' and yet they may be aware that day-to-day living requires more effort and that they do not have their usual zest for life; or it may be a very severe depression, which is obvious even to the unsophisticated, and which may require psychiatric in-patient treatment. Between these two extremes are patients who become aware of feelings of relative sadness and depression, who may confront their family doctor and be referred to the hospital out-patient clinic for psychiatric treatment. In this type of depression, the mood of dejection is greater than could be anticipated from the patient's circumstances. There is a striking loss of in-itiative, and life becomes a burden to the patient; his usual con-fidence deserts him and he may express feelings of inferiority. Decisions, which would have been taken almost without thought in the past, become an effort and, if there is marked anxiety associated with the depression (as quite often occurs), agitation may be a striking feature of the patient's mental state. Irritability and tear-fulness may occur, particularly when there is this marked degree of associated anxiety.

Thinking and activity may be affected. In many instances, mobility is reduced and, in an extreme case, activity and thinking may be slowed to such an extent that the patient may appear to be in a stupor. However, if marked associated anxiety is present, there may be pressure of thinking, with thoughts crowding in on one another and consequently the patient may be overactive.

In addition, the patient may show disturbance in thought content and may even experience delusions. These may be delusions of guilt; for example, he may feel he has committed such a terrible sin that he cannot be forgiven. It is usually not too difficult to establish that there is no factual foundation for this belief, although he will be temporarily unable to accept reassurance, on account of his illness.

In the older age group we may see delusions of poverty, in which the patient believes that he must scrimp and save, as he cannot afford even the essentials of daily living, although in reality he has adequate resources. (This particular form of delusional belief is rare in adolescence.) Again, a patient may believe that he has an incurable disease, such as cancer, or be preoccupied with some disturbance of bodily health or function (hypochondriacal delusions). Obsessional thinking, in which an idea keeps recurring until the patient is unable to resist it, although he recognises that it is ridiculous, may sometimes be a feature of a depressive illness. (Obsessional thinking will be discussed in more detail in the section on obsessional neurosis—*see* Chapter 12. The difference is, that in this instance the obsessional symptoms disappear when the depression is relieved.) The behavioural component of this, the compulsive act, when the patient feels he must carry out certain acts although he believes them to be silly, responds similarly to improvement in the depression.

Sometimes a depressive patient experiences de-personalisation, in which he feels he has changed in comparison with his former self, so that he no longer acknowledges himself as a personality. His actions appear to be automatic and it is as if he were observing himself from outside.

The most seriously depressed patients feel that life is not worth living and will contemplate self-harm. It is said that one patient in six, diagnosed as suffering from manic-depressive illness, can be expected eventually to take his own life. Apart from those who make a successful suicide attempt there are others who have been interrupted in the attempt, but who nevertheless continue to feel that life is not worth living. This last is such an important symptom in adolescence that it will be discussed specially in the next chapter.

*   *   *

There is evidence of a close link between the manic-type and the depressive-type of affective disorder. Some patients have manic episodes succeeded, or preceded, by depressive episodes. In general, depressive episodes are said to be more common than manic episodes, but in an interesting study in Norway, Dr. T. Olsen examined the case records of adult patients with a proven manic-depressive illness who had been admitted to a psychiatric hospital under the age of 19. In this series, he found that a patient's first admission was more likely to be on account of a manic episode, so it may be that in adolescence manic episodes are more common, although as I have mentioned, both elation and dejection are quite likely to be unrecognised as illness in adolescents, when present to a mild degree. Dejection does occur in normal adolescents, but it is not usually prolonged and, as indicated in Chapter 3, Dr. Masterson found in a controlled study that the depth of depression was usually more serious in his patient-group than in the control-group, and suicidal thoughts did not occur in the control group. In adult psychiatry, the marked physical features, in particular sleep disturbance, contribute to the establishment of a correct diagnosis, but in the author's experience, sleep disturbance is less common and more likely to be atypical in teenagers. Many depressed adolescents, instead of waking early, will spend half the day in bed, and it is the lack of initiative in contract to the boisterousness of the normal juvenile which excites comment.

The classical manic-depressive illness which has just been described rarely occurs before puberty, and although it does occur in adolescence, its onset is most common in the third decade of life. It tends to be more common in females than in males, and attacks are more likely to develop in the late spring and early summer, with a further peak in the autumn. Depressive illness typically runs a periodic course, a depressive episode being followed by a period of normality of variable duration, followed by a further period of illness which might be depression or mania, again to be succeeded by a period of normality. Until recently, the main aim was to treat the individual episode and, in at least two-thirds of cases, the psychiatrist could expect at least reasonable success, but with newer methods of treatment, to be discussed below, in some patients it is now actually possible to reduce the number of attacks.

Dr. Olsen's follow-up study on manic-depressive illness in patients who had had their first attack before the age of 19 years, demonstrated that attacks were liable to persist or recur over a two-year period, but after that the patient might remain well until early adult life, when recurrence was likely.

Aetiological factors

The cause of affective disorder is not known. However, from the results of twin studies, there is evidence of a genetic predisposition to this type of illness, but just why the illness takes so long to become manifest and what possible precipitating factors there may be, have still to be worked out. Early-life experience of patients who develop depressive illnesses in adult life have been examined in detail; it was postulated that loss of a parent due to bereavement in childhood might be related to the subsequent development of an affective illness. Results in this field have tended to be controversial. Separation from parents in childhood, for reasons other than death, have not been found to occur more commonly in patients with affective illness than in the general population.

The personality of the patient with a depressive illness has been commented on in relation to the outlook, although this has not been studied in as much detail as might have been expected, in view of the weight put upon it by some authors. Many observers have commented on the good prognosis in relation to a 'good previous personality'. The so-called cyclothymic temperament has some relationship with manic-depressive illness. In this, individuals tend to appear rather dejected in their general outlook on life or show mild elation with considerable zest for life; either of these moods may predominate, or there may be a fluctuation from one to the other. In general, patients who develop a manic-depressive illness appear to be rather conscientious and reliable.

Physical aspects

1. It is recognised that people with a 'pyknic' body build (i.e. possessing a stocky physique), more frequently suffer from affective disorders than would be expected from their numbers in the general population.
2. Following a severe attack of influenza, or sometimes other viral infections, the normal post-infective depression can become prolonged and requires treatment in its own right as a depressive illness.

Biochemical aspects

One group of drugs which may have a beneficial effect on depressed mood are known as mono-amine oxidase inhibitors,

because of the inactivating or inhibiting effect they exert on an enzyme known as mono-amine oxidase. This enzyme has the function, as its name implies, of oxidising certain chemical substances
known as mono-amines. Mono-amines thought to be important in
brain function are 5-hydroxytryptamine (5-HT) or Serotonin and
noradrenaline. From animal studies, it was observed that Reserpine—a drug used in the early days of the medical treatment of
high blood pressure—tended to deplete the 5-HT and noradrenaline stores in the brain, but this effect could be prevented by
treatment with a mono-amine oxidase inhibitor, or a member of
another group of drugs known as the tricyclic anti-depressants.
These observations have stimulated much research work on brain
metabolism, although as yet the final answer regarding the
biochemistry of mood is still far from being found.

Treatment
According to the severity of the patient's depression or elation,
treatment will be undertaken by the patient's family doctor, or at a
psychiatric outpatient clinic at a hospital, or as an in-patient, and
will consist of:

1. Physical methods of treatment.
2. Environmental changes where indicated.

The drug treatment of depression
The treatment of this form of illness is possibly the most satisfactory form of psychiatric treatment available today. Since the 1960s,
it has been carried out most usually with anti-depressant drugs.
There are two main groups of anti-depressant drugs:

1. The tricyclic anti-depressants.
2. The monoamine oxidase inhibitors.

The detailed description of the actions and side effects of these
drugs is given in Chapter 18.

Electro-convulsive therapy (E.C.T.)
Before anti-depressant drugs became available, E.C.T. was used
extensively and successfully in the treatment of depression; again
the details of the type of treatment are taken up in Chapter 18.

Anti-depressant drugs may be combined with E.C.T. and frequently reduce the number of treatments required.

Leucotomy

In intractable cases in which the patient has recurrent episodes of illness which fail to respond to conventional methods of treatment, brain surgery, known as leucotomy, may have to be considered. However, with improved methods of treatment and the use of lithium, to be described later, leucotomy is rarely undertaken, and is most unlikely to be considered in the adolescent age period.

The drug treatment of manic illness

The drug treatment of elation is less specific than that of depression. Again, two main groups of drugs are used to control the patient's over-activity and uninhibited behaviour. These are: 1, the phenothiazine group of drugs, and 2, the butyrophenone group of drugs.

Phenothiazine

The best known drug of the *phenothiazine* group is chlorpromazine (Largactil) first introduced in 1952. Other types of phenothiazines have an alteration in their molecular structure and they are classified according to their chemical structure.

Butyrophenone

The *butyrophenone* group of drugs are also major tranquillisers and may be given orally or by injection. Like the phenothiazines they have an impressive effect on disturbed behaviour, overactivity, excitement and aggressiveness, but even more than the phenothiazines they are likely to produce marked Parkinsonian features and so must be accompanied by the use of anti-Parkinsonian drugs. The exact way in which these drugs act is unknown but it would appear that they damp down symptoms rather than attack the cause of the illness. Again the reader is referred to Chapter 18 for a detailed description of these drugs.

Lithium carbonate

This was introduced to psychiatry for the treatment of mania in the 1940s, but due to serious side-effects it fell into disrepute. However, recently it has been reintroduced as a valuable drug to prevent recurrence of manic or depressive episodes. Undoubtedly, lithium is a dangerous drug and patients taking it must remain under regular medical supervision whilst they are on it. The dose of lithium is that required to maintain the blood level at a therapeutic level. This is between 0·6 and 1·4 millimols per litre. Toxic symptoms appear when the blood level rises to 2·0 millimols per litre, so it would seem that the therapeutic level and the toxic level are fairly close.

The use of lithium has been a marked advance in the treatment of manic-depressive illness and in the prevention of recurrences, but the indications for the use of this drug and its ultimate place in the management of the illness have still to be worked out.

General management

Many depressed adolescents become further dejected during treatment related to their primary depression and the inertia with which they have had to contend for so long, so that they very much need a humane psychological approach as well as any specific drug-treatment.

When depression is most severe and the patient feels that he will never be cured it is legitimate to reassure him that the situation will improve with treatment. He may think that he will never be able to achieve his ambitions. In marked degrees of depression, the patient will have to give up work or school and in the most severe type, bed-rest may be beneficial. In mild depression, or as a severe depression begins to improve, environmental factors contributing to the mental state should be examined, and discussed with the patient. Appropriate action should then be taken, but it is important for all those involved with the patient, and particularly for relatives, to recognise that *the environmental stresses may be the result of the patient's inability to cope with everyday life and not the cause of his illness.*

Patients must be discouraged from making major decisions whilst they are ill, whether it be depression or hypomania. Some patients feel that if they could just change their job, their school or their house everything would be all right, but in fact it is the patient's mental state which is wrong and not the circumstances. The manic patient may feel particularly erotic as a result of his illness and decide that he would like to marry after the briefest of acquaintance: again, he should be discouraged. Manic or depressed patients whose illness is sufficiently severe for them to be admitted to hospital should be advised that no major decisions should be taken until they have been living in the community again for six to twelve months.

It is at this stage also that assessment of the patient's personality becomes important. The more inadequate patient is likely to be overwhelmed by his symptoms and the effect of the illness, whereas the energetic, conscientious patient will be more able to cope with this.

The psychiatrist used to treating adult patients may become impatient because the response to treatment, in teenagers who have episodes of depression or hypomania, may be less dramatic than in the older patient. However, correctly diagnosed and treated, the outcome of manic-depressive illness is likely to be satisfactory to patient and therapist alike, even when delays do occur.

REFERENCES AND FURTHER READING

Anderson, E. W. and Trethowan, W. H., Chapter 11, 'Affective Disorder' in *Psychiatry*. Ballière Tindall, 3rd Ed., 1973.

Coppen, A. and Walk, A. *Recent Developments in Affective Disorders*. Publ. for Royal Medico-Psychological Assoc. by Headley Brothers Ltd., 1968.

Olsen, T. 'A follow-up study of Manic-depressive patients whose first attack occurred before the age of 19 years'. Act. Psychiat. Scan. 1961 Suppl. 162 p. 145.

Registrar General. *A Glossary of Mental Disorder*. Prepared by Sub-committee on Classification of Mental Disorders of the Registrar General's Advisory Committee on Medical Nomenclature and statistics. H.M.S.O., 1968.

Sim, M. Chapter 12 'Affective Disorders,' in *A Guide to Psychiatry*. Churchill Livingstone. 3rd Ed., 1974.

Slater, E. and Roth, M. Chapter 4 'Affective Disorders,' *Clinical Psychiatry*. Ballière Tindall and Cassell, 3rd Ed., 1969.

7 Self-harm in adolescence

The suicidal attempt has been defined as 'any deliberate act of self-injury apparently aimed at self-destruction, however, vague an attempt or trivial the danger'.

CLINICAL FEATURES

In the last decade, there has been a marked increase in the number of patients admitted to the medical wards of general hospitals as a consequence of 'self-poisoning'. Mistakes do occur occasionally, but the majority of these admissions are the result of intentional self-administration of an overdose of drugs. Death may occur and this will be discussed later, but the majority of young persons receiving medical aid at an early stage recover and an approach should then be made to the psychiatrist to assess the patient's need for psychiatric help. Ideally, the patient should be seen whilst still an in-patient, but he may be given an early out-patient appointment instead. The disadvantage of this is that there is no guarantee that the appointment will be kept.

The episode of self-harm is merely a symptom and the cause must be determined. The sort of situation which may arise is one where, for example, a teenager has been playing truant from school, realises that the non-attendance has come to light and that shortly the school will be making contact with his family. He may be ashamed of having let the family down, of the disgrace he is bringing to his relatives and decides that life is no longer worth living. Impulsively, he may then go to the bathroom cupboard and find a bottle of aspirin, or a relative's tranquillisers or sleeping tablets, and take the lot. At that moment, he feels that he would be better off dead. Depending on the teenager's actions, the type of tablet taken and the presence or absence of the family in the house at the time of the ingestion of the tablets, the situation may or may not be recognised for what it is. A particularly dangerous episode is when the tablets are taken at night as the teenager is going to bed and it is only when he cannot be awakened for school next morning that it is recognised that something is amiss: in unfortunate circumstances he may be found dead.

In a more favourable situation, the teenager may be roused and get up, but then will be noticed to be staggering around the house, or he may even slump to the floor. Occasionally, after taking an overdose of aspirin, the young person may waken vomiting in the middle of the night and this may rouse another member of the family. Once the situation is recognised the patient may be taken to the Casualty Department of a local hospital, either on a relative's own initiative or at the instigation of a general practitioner. Here a doctor will try to find out what tablets have been taken and the patient may have a gastric lavage (stomach washout or 'stomach pump') to remove any tablets which may be lying unabsorbed in the stomach. Further treatment to counteract the effects of the drugs already absorbed will be carried out as indicated. The tablets most commonly taken are sleeping tablets, nerve tablets (tranquillisers), or aspirin-like tablets.

Once the essential physical treatment has been undertaken, the doctor will attempt to find out from the patient (if well enough) and from the relatives why he took the tablets. It is whilst the patient is recovering from the after-effects of the overdose that the psychiatrist is likely to be involved and he will want to know why the patient has been playing truant from school, or whatever other problem appears to be uppermost. It may be that assessment of intelligence and academic achievement, a change of school, or other intervention in the environment, would be appropriate in such a case, and moves can be made to initiate such procedures.

After recovery, some patients regret having taken the overdose and feel that they have let themselves down even further and then they need help in facing the community again. This is particularly the case with school children, especially if the overdose was taken *at* school and other pupils are aware of the reason for the patient's admission to hospital. With support, the teenager can usually accept that, at worst, it will be a 'nine days wonder' and that the sooner the situation is faced the easier it will be. Obviously, the reaction of the staff at school will be important. Usually it is best for them to accept that the episode, even if it did occur on school premises, is being dealt with elsewhere and not to badger the returning pupil with questions. When the overdose occurred elsewhere and outside the school hours, should the school be told? Obviously, this can only be done if the patient and his parents agree and if it is felt that it is in the youngster's best interest. The school medical officer will usually be informed (doctor-to-doctor information is confidential) and he or she will often know the particular school well enough to anticipate what reaction the knowledge may evoke. Even today, some schools over-react to such information. In several instances known to the author, the head teachers have been reluctant to have back to school a pupil who has taken an overdose, even though the tablets were not swallowed on school premises, and were taken out of school hours and for a reason totally unrelated to the school. On account of reactions such as this, one cannot recommend unreservedly to parents that it would be in the child's best interests for the school to be informed, but each case should be judged on its own merits.

Where school is the main problem, the reason for the episode of self-harm may be quite clear and the problem may resolve spontaneously or with help. Sometimes a teenager who is unhappy at home may take a similar overdose and receive the same investigation. In such a setting the doctor would have to decide whether it was appropriate for the teenager to return to the home environment. It may be that, having talked over the difficulties in the home situation with the patient and key figures there, the teenager will be under less pressure and may safely return home. Under different circumstances, it may become apparent that the teenager is too vulnerable to cope with the pressures or stress of a given environment. Then involvement of the local authority Social Services

Department is important, so that the situation can be reviewed and, if necessary, the youngster admitted to the care of the local authority. Only too often one sees teenagers returning home to an unhappy situation and being readmitted to hospital two weeks later, having taken a further and sometimes more serious overdose. The key question then that those involved in the assessment of adolescents, and indeed all patients, must ask is 'What has been achieved by the episode of self-harm?' If the problems which resulted in the overdose remain, ways must be sought to ameliorate the situation or, alternatively, to remove the patient from the particular stress for a period of assessment at least.

The above are fairly common examples of the background to hospital admission following a suicidal attempt in an impulsive youngster who may have a low tolerance of frustration. However, another person taking an overdose of tablets may do so because of a serious depression as discussed in Chapter 6. As a result of a depressive illness, the patient may feel that life is not worth living and be unable to see a future for himself. Treatment will be that of the underlying depression as has already been outlined and inpatient treatment may be required if the depression is severe.

Occasionally, the reason behind the suicidal attempt is not at all clear. The episode itself may be out of character for the patient and then the question of a schizophrenic illness may arise (see Chapter 5). In such patients, a suicidal attempt is most likely to occur in the early stage of the illness, when some insight is preserved. The patient is bewildered and perplexed by the disintegration of his thinking, emotions and personality. Some schizophrenics may make a suicidal attempt in response to hallucinatory voices urging them to harm themselves. Schizophrenia is now considered to be a fairly rare cause of attempted self-harm in adolescence, but obviously it is an important one to recognise.

CONTRIBUTORY FACTORS

It has been suggested that the overall incidence of suicidal attempts in an urban community is eight to ten times that of successful suicide, but during adolescence the proportion of attempts is much higher. There is a considerable literature on attempted suicide in adult life and a growing number of reports on suicidal attempts in adolescence. The majority of these are retrospective and are based on studies of records made before the passing of the Suicide Act of 1961, or on series of cases known to the police in a given city. Reports from the United States and Scandinavia are perhaps more helpful and are fairly consistent in their findings. Adolescent females attempt self-harm more frequently than males, in the order of 5 to 1 or 6 to 1, in contrast to the sex ratio of 3 to 1 quoted for adults.

Self-harm is rare under the age of 10, but the number reported rises in the 10 to 14 age group. There is then a marked increase in the 15 to 19 age group, but the majority of suicidal attempts are in the third decade of life (20 to 29 years). The infrequency of self-harm before the age of ten deserves comment. No satisfactory explanation of this has been put forward, but two possibilities merit consideration:

1. As discussed in Chapter 2, in the first decade of life thinking is concrete and it is only in the second decade of life that young people begin to think in more abstract terms. In relation to this alteration in thinking they also become more introspective. Could this be a factor in suicidal attempts commencing after the age of ten years?

2. Quite a number of studies have now been carried out on the development of the child's concept of death. Overall, it would appear that in the first five years of life death is regarded as a departure. Life continues elsewhere, albeit under changed conditions and separation is the most important factor. It is only in those of 9 years and over that the universality of death is realised and the fact that it is the end of corporeal life. Some workers have attempted to link this maturation of the concept of death with intellectual maturation. To an extent, these views have been borne out by the experience of those working with children on paediatric wards who suffer from leukaemia and other malignant diseases, where again, only towards the end of the first decade of life does fear of death become prominent.

Kessel, studying the problem of overdose in Edinburgh, estimated that, in a single year, more than one out of every five hundred Edinburgh girls aged 15 to 19 years poisoned herself. He suggested that the high teenage rate of self-harm in girls may be the

female counterpart of delinquency. He also put forward the
hypothesis that young married women, although fully engaged in
their normal function of mothering and running a house, may be
emotionally isolated. Until recently, they had been experiencing an
active social life and had not had time to adjust to the confines of
domesticity. His formulation is not tenable, as many younger
adolescents who are still at school or are gainfully employed may
have a fairly involved social life.

In adult studies, the association of attempted suicide with the
more deprived section of the community has been commented on,
but this has not been described as a feature of self-harm in
adolescents.

Studies of adult attempted suicide make comment on the high
proportion of suicidal attempts associated with serious depression.
Early studies of self-harm in adolescence in America suggested
that schizophrenia was a more common cause than depression
in adolescents, but later studies have failed to support these
findings.

As with teenagers presenting with conduct disorders, a disorganised home background is not uncommon, and there may be a
history of deliquency in the family. Youngsters with immature, impulsive, personality traits who over-react to minor stress may make
a suicidal attempt. Symptoms of dejection, restlessness, boredom,
sexual promiscuity, running away and truancy from school are
common antecedents to the attempt itself and are of particular
significance when they seem out of character.

Emotional features focussed on in the literature include anger,
for example 'They'll be sorry when I'm dead', depression or dissatisfaction. The teenager with a vulnerable self-esteem may be unable to cope with a fear of failure, or of letting the family down.
Associated with such fears may be anxiety about what other people
may think or do. Sometimes the adolescent in need of help may use
the overdose as a signal of distress to draw attention to his
problems. At other times there may be a deliberate attempt to
manipulate a situation to his own advantage. Often a combination
of factors such as these will be found.

Precipitating factors involve conflict in the home, for example
over domestic chores, late nights, trendy dress, choice of friends, or
school matters such as homework.

MANAGEMENT

At one period, it was customary to expend considerable energy on assessing the 'seriousness' of the suicidal attempt. In the author's view this is dangerous in the adolescent age group and efforts should be aimed instead at deciding on the factors contributing to the episode of self-harm and helping to ensure that a further suicidal attempt does not ensue. It is quite wrong to assume in all cases where the attempt has not endangered life that, the patient did not have a genuine wish to die. The knowledge required to ensure a fatal outcome may require a degree of sophistication which the teenager does not have at his command. However, it *is* true that the teenager acting impulsively is more likely to be reacting to environmental stress, whereas the teenager making a premeditated attempt, carefully planned and carried out, is more likely to be seriously depressed. In either case the psychiatrist may feel that the patient requires observation as an in-patient in a psychiatric ward. Over the age of 16, the patient will give his own consent. Under the age of 16, the consent of both parent and patient should be sought. However, if the parents do not take the suicidal attempt seriously, or if the patient seems fully intent on killing himself and feels foiled by his lack of success, this consent may be withheld. If the psychiatrist is of the opinion that such a patient is seriously intending to kill himself and this opinion is supported by another doctor and a social worker, the patient should be transferred to a psychiatric ward for observation under Section 25 of the Mental Health Act 1959. A patient admitted to hospital under such a Section is termed a 'formal patient', in contradistinction to the 'informal' patient, who is over 16 and has given his own consent to treatment.

Every suicidal attempt *must* be taken seriously. At the least, the attempt was an effort at some form of communication and this must be appreciated by careful attention to its antecedents. In many instances it is also important that parents or other key figures in the environment should be aware of the message, as this may well reduce the risk of repetition. Obviously, parental anxiety will be high when a patient who has attempted to harm himself returns home. This should be explained to the patient and the parents before the former is discharged. The patient has to appreciate that he must gradually regain the trust and confidence of his parents.

Parents must be encouraged to take a sympathetic attitude, and yet at the same time should be aware that, with a particularly manipulative youngster, there is a risk that they will be blackmailed with the threat of a further suicidal attempt if his wishes are thwarted. This is unhealthy, but the approach should be one of constructive anticipation rather than trying to adopt a moral attitude to the episode.

Is psychiatric treatment of value in these cases? A study from King's College Hospital published in 1972 has suggested that it is. Patients who made suicidal attempts were followed up and those not referred for psychiatric assessment were compared with these subsequently attending a psychiatric out-patient clinic. It was found that those who did not have psychiatric supervision were more likely to make a further attempt. Unfortunately, the information provided by the investigators is not quite complete and it may be that those who were not referred for psychiatric treatment were regarded as having a worse prognosis and this was why they were not sent to the psychiatrist in the first instance!

COMPLETED SUICIDE

Death in adolescence is rare and the factors contributing to it have been changing in recent years. In the United Kingdom and the United States of America, death from natural causes has been superseded by deaths from violence, particularly street-traffic accidents, as a leading cause of mortality in the adolescent population. Malignant neoplasm and diseases of the nervous system and cardiovascular system are next in order and suicide is now becoming a significant cause of death. In some areas of America suicide is now fourth in rank as the cause of death in males aged 15 to 19 years and the suicide rate is continuing to increase significantly in this group.

In 1967, Dr. Reginald Lourie, reviewing the subject of suicide and suicidal attempts in children and adolescents, described a periodic shift of emphasis in placing the blame for child suicide. From 1880 to 1900, the chief culprits were said to be the trashy novels and romantic sentimental stories of the times. From 1900 to 1915, the tendency in the majority of reports was to place the blame on the educational system and from 1915 to 1936, the emphasis was on constitutional factors. It is only in the last thirty-odd years that there has been speculation on the deeper underlying motivations of children wanting to die.

At the end of the eighteenth century, Caspar reported from Prussia on a few child suicides for the years 1788 to 1797. Since then, the figures have shown an irregular increase in the number of cases in the Western world. At the beginning of the present century, there was a world-wide increase in the child suicide rate, the rate being particularly high in Prussia and Russia. Bakwin quotes that in Saxony from 1903 to 1907 the suicide rate in the 10 to 15 age group was 5·3 per 10,000 for males and 2·6 per 10,000 for females, and in the 16 to 19 age group it rose to 34·1 per 10,000 for males and 19·2 per 10,000 for females. These rates are ten times as high as comparable figures for the United States of America in 1954. It is notable that, even at the beginning of this century, the rates in predominantly Catholic areas of Prussia were only a fraction of those in other areas.

Japan currently has the highest rate of teenage suicide. Whilst in adults its rate is comparable to that in Austria, Denmark and Switzerland, in adolescents it has more than twice the rate in any other country. The incidence remains high in Japan until 25 years of age and then decreases, rising again after the age of 60. This picture is similar for both sexes. Another interesting feature is that whereas in most other countries the male/female ratio for successful suicide is 3 to 1 or 4 to 1, in Japan in the younger age group the ratio is 1·7 to 1. In fact, the suicide rate for Japanese girls is higher than the rate for males in all other countries and for both sexes the higher rate for urban areas observed elsewhere is not seen in Japan. Also, in contradistinction to other countries where suicide rates continued to fall after the Second World War, until 1955, in Japan the rate began to increase as soon as the war ended and the rate had quadrupled by 1960, when it started to decline. One explanation put forward to explain this difference was that statistics were inaccurate in the War years, but this does not seem to provide a convincing reason. In recent years, it is probable that with increasing Western influences in Japan, suicidal attempts have declined as traditional influences have become less.

A psychiatrist working with adults attempts to distinguish between those patients who have a clear desire to die and those who attempt suicide in order to draw attention to the difficulties which they are experiencing, the aim of the latter being to obtain help and not death. As mentioned above, it is doubtful if this concept is tenable when assessing the nature of suicidal attempts in adolescents. The author has had the opportunity to look at a number of Coroner's records, of the last decade, where a verdict of suicide in adolescence has been recorded. Of the 46 records studied there were 28 males and 18 females aged 13 to 20 years. Seven (5 females and 2 males) were married. For the method used *see* Table 3.

TABLE 3
Method of Suicide Related to Sex

Method		Male	Female	Total
Coal gas poisoning		15	12	27
Overdose of drugs:		7	4	11
Barbituates	7			
Cyanide	2			
Antidepressants	1			
Tranquillisers	1			
Strangulation		1	1	2
Hanging		2	1	3
Fall from a height		1		1
Firearm		1		1
Threw self under train		1		1
		28	18	46
Suicide note left		5	7	12

As might have been anticipated, the violent methods were usually employed by males. The precipitating factors in many of these suicide bids were similar; for example, 11 occurred directly after a row with an all-important boy-/girl-friend, in 6 police action was pending, and in 2 cases parents were about to learn that the individual concerned had been truanting from school. In only 5 cases could a definite diagnosis of psychiatric illness be sustained on the evidence available and two of these were hospital in-patients at the time of death. In 3 cases, the suspicion of pregnancy had just been confirmed and in only one of these was it an extra-marital pregnancy. Case records showed that 6 had made previous suicidal threats and 9 had made previous attempts. It is interesting that there was a family history of overdose of drugs in two instances.

Most studies of successful adolescent suicide come from the United States of America where, for both sexes, the use of firearms and explosives is the most common method of suicide, followed by hanging and strangulation in boys and poisoning in girls. As with adults, there is often a previous history of an unsuccessful suicidal bid.

In the case of suicide, there is no one afterwards who can truly describe the background to the episode. However, the evidence that is available suggests that those in the younger age group who commit suicide come from a background which is very similar to those attempting self-harm, in terms of social disorganisation and distress. Given the right facilities, it is possible to delineate those groups of adolescents who are at greatly increased risk of attempting or committing suicide. However, it would demand enormous resources, that are not available, to institute an effective preventive service and so far there has been little obvious success in those centres which have tried to set up such a service. At present our involvement is too often *after* the event: with timely intervention the event may not be fatal. Despite the problems involved, this is an area worthy of very considerable study and effort; its complexity should not deter; nor should it conceal the great amount of human suffering involved, where a young person feels sufficiently desperate even to think seriously of harming himself.

REFERENCES AND FURTHER READING

Bakwin, H. 'Suicide in Children and Adolescents.' J. Paed., 1957, *50*, 749.

Connell, P. 'Suicidal Attempts in Childhood and Adolescence.' Chapter XVII in *Modern Perspectives in Child Psychiatry*. Ed. J. G. Howell. Oliver & Boyd, 1965.

Greer, S. and Bagley, C., 'The Effect of Psychiatric Intervention in Attempted Suicide.' B.M.J., 1971, *1*, 310.

Kessel, N. 'Self Poisoning I & II.' B.M.J., 1965, ii, 1265, 1336.

Lourie, R. 'Suicide and Attempted Suicide in Children and Adolescents.' Texas Medicine, 1967, *63*, 58.

Otto, U. 'Suicidal Attempts made by Children.' Act. Paed. Scan., 1966, *55*, 64.

Otto, U. 'Suicidal Acts by Children and Adolescents Follow-up study.'
  Act. Psych. Scan., Suppl. 233.
Shaffer, D. 'Suicide in Childhood and Early Adolescence.' J. Child
  Psychol. Psychiat., 1974, *15*, 275.
Toolan, J. M. 'Suicide and Suicidal Attempts in Children and
  Adolescents.' Am. J. Psychiat., 1961, *118*, 719.

8 Drug abuse

A *drug* is a chemical substance, natural or synthetic, which has an action on body metabolism. This action may be helpful or harmful. *Pharmacology* is the study of the action of drugs on the animal organism and *medicinal therapeutics* is the science and art of using the action of drugs in the treatment of disease. Until this century, the number of drugs known to man, with a potent therapeutic action, was limited, but during this century, many powerful drugs have been discovered to aid in the control of disease. Readers will be aware of the antibiotics which help to control infection. Nowadays, some diseases of the endocrine glands (glands of internal secretion, such as the thyroid gland and pituitary gland) can be controlled by medication; for example, the young diabetic can now live a relatively normal life, provided he has a daily injection of insulin. Many epileptics (people who suffer from recurring episodes in which they may lose consciousness—*see* Chapter 16) are able to lead satisfying lives if they take drugs to control their attacks; these drugs, known as anticonvulstants, have to be taken regularly over a long period. For reasons like this, there is a small group of teenagers for whom drug-taking is beneficial and may, indeed, be essential for life and health. (It is an unfortunate sign of the times to report that epileptics have occasionally been, mistakenly, regarded as misusing drugs and attempts have been made to wean them off

95

their medically-prescribed anti-convulsant tablets, by well-meaning but misguided adults.)

The effects of appropriately prescribed drugs are largely beneficial but, inevitably, there are undesirable side effects and often the therapeutic dose is very close to the level at which toxic effects may appear. By and large, adolescents are healthy and rarely have to seek medical advice. If an adolescent has a headache or cough, he may consult his local chemist for an appropriate pain-killer or cough-mixture, or he may select his own medication from the shelf at the local supermarket without prior consultation. The re-introduction of the National Health Service prescription charge has encouraged self-medication in many groups of people.

As an earlier generation was preoccupied with bowel habit and consumed large quantities of laxatives, so the present population is concerned with insomnia and nervous tension and there has been an increase in the prescription of sleeping tablets and tranquillisers in the last decade. These drugs act through the nervous system where they exert a sedative effect. The opiate group of drugs, which includes heroin, morphine and the synthetic substance pethidine, is used medically for the relief of severe pain after operations or in cases of serious, painful illness. These substances also have an effect on the mood state and the level of consciousness. Another group of drugs are 'pep pills', or stimulants, which were popular with students who used them to help to keep themselves awake to study and with long-distance drivers, air-line pilots, mountaineers and athletes for similar reasons, until their use was discouraged. Before the present anti-depressant drugs became available, these stimulants (usually amphetamines) were prescribed by doctors for patients because of their energising effect on the central nervous system. With continued use, the body becomes tolerant of substances influencing the central nervous system, so that it is necessary to increase the dose of the drug to obtain the same effect and this was found to be tragically true of both opiates and pep pills.

After the First World War, there was some concern about drug abuse in this country, but drug dependence was in the main confined to those who had access to drugs, for example, doctors, nurses and pharmacists, or those who became addicted in the course of medical treatment. Young people were rarely involved.

Over the past fifteen years, drug abuse has become an increasing problem, and the striking feature of this has been the number of young people under twenty-five years who have resorted to drugs. The importance of a uniform—some outward and visible identifying sign—in helping teenagers to identify with each other, was mentioned in Chapter 2, but latterly it has seemed that 'trendy gear' is insufficient and so behavioural requirements have become more marked, for example sexual prowess, some delinquent acts, and, in some instances, drug abuse. As in the high-delinquency areas of cities, where one does not move up the gang hierarchy until one has been to a juvenile remand centre, so, in other localities, referral to the regional drug addiction centre has become an important way of enhancing prestige and, consequently, drug abuse has become a serious concern to those interested in the welfare of juveniles.

DEFINITION

The problem of drug addiction has been the concern of the World Health Organisation's Expert Committee on drug dependence, and in a report published in 1957 this committee attempted to distinguish between drug addiction and drug habituation. However, this distinction led to practical difficulties and a further report in 1964 recommended the use of the comprehensive term 'drug dependence', defined as 'A state, sometimes psychic (psychological) and sometimes also physical, resulting from the interaction between a living organism and a drug, characterised by behavioural and other responses that always includes a compulsion to take the drug on a continuous or periodic basis in order to experience its psychic effects and sometimes to avoid the discomfort of its absence'. The W.H.O. report went on to say that tolerance to the drug might or might not be present and that a person might be dependent on more than one drug.

When working with a given teenager, it may be difficult to decide if all the criteria required to meet the definition of drug dependence are present, but one may have ample evidence of abuse of drugs. Recently, this latter term has come to be used a good deal. It is important that the terms 'drug dependence' or 'drug abuse' should not be used lightly. For example, the teenager who takes a couple of extra aspirins because of a blinding headache should certainly not be labelled as a drug abuser.

When considering drug abuse, two factors have to be taken into account:

1. The drug.
2. The drug-taker.

The drug

A variety of drugs is abused by adolescents, sometimes alone and sometimes in combination.

Alcohol remains the commonest means of addiction in our culture. It is easily available and its use is accepted by many, to the extent that social drinking may appear a desirable habit. There is growing concern about under-age drinking and the increasing number of young alcoholics being admitted to hospital for treatment. Review of legislation on the age at which alcohol may be consumed in a public bar—now age 18—was undertaken recently and it was decided not to recommend a lowering of the age.

In certain occupations, exposure to alcohol is difficult to avoid. Alcoholism is a well-recognised occupational hazard for commercial travellers and bartenders, for example, but, as with other forms of drug abuse, factors other than occupation are now influencing the picture. In the East, where a contemplative way of life is valued, opium-smoking has long been recognised and to some extent it substitutes for the alcohol of the Western world. It is interesting that, in the United States, Chinese immigrants have a low rate of opium addiction.

When the present increase in drug abuse began, it became apparent that young people in London tended to look down on individuals who indulged in alcohol which dulled the senses, as they preferred something which would excite them and give them 'kicks' and thus many of them took pep pills. A fairly typical pattern emerged in the early nineteen-sixties. Initially, a teenager might just take a pep pill as an experiment, in the same way as an adolescent of an earlier generation tried a cigarette in a quiet corner, but then for some the 'week-ender' stage followed. This was when a pep pill was taken at a party to keep the teenager from feeling drowsy, so that he could continue to enjoy himself into the small hours. At one stage, pep pills were handed around in many of the coffee bars in London and the provinces. Most of them contained the drug

amphetamine, or one of its derivatives, often combined with a barbiturate drug. The common names for these included 'blues', 'black
bombers' and 'green bombers'. Perhaps fortunately, many young
people dabbling with drugs do not progress beyond this point, at
which the actual taking of the drug is only a small part of their
satisfaction.

In the next stage, the teenager who is becoming 'hooked' starts
taking larger and larger numbers of tablets and it would appear
that it is often the taking of the tablet which then provides satisfaction. If the tablet is not available, the individual feels let down, tired
and unhappy. At this stage, drug taking may still be confined to the
week-ends, but by Monday morning it may be difficult to get out of
bed to work, and so it becomes necessary to take a tablet in order
to face the day. Initially, this is confined to Monday mornings, but
gradually it spreads to other days of the week and with each day
the dose is increased and it becomes harder to get a sufficient supply of tablets. Then the young drug-taker resorts to various devices,
legal and illegal, to obtain further supplies of tablets. This may involve stealing money, breaking and entering doctor's surgeries, and
stealing National Health Service prescription pads in order to write
out their own prescriptions. In the days when it was legitimate to
prescribe amphetamines, the number of tablets prescribed would
sometimes be altered on a legitimate prescription. Also, many
'kindly' fat ladies would acquire 'slimming pills' from their family
doctor and would then sell them on the black market to desperate
teenagers.

Once he is seriously abusing drugs, a teenager loses control of
his behaviour. His work record deteriorates, as it is difficult for him
to get up in the morning. (In fact, this is often one of the first signs
that a parent can recognise.) Family life becomes disrupted and the
teenager frequently leaves home at this stage. He may be subject to
increasing irritability and outbursts of aggression and become involved in petty crime.

In the past, a teenager who was abusing amphetamine might
then begin to experiment with other drugs, such as marijuana (cannabis) also known as Indian hemp, hashish or 'pot', sometimes
graduating thereafter to what are called the hard drugs, for example
cocaine and heroin.

Until a few years ago, this pattern was fairly typical of the way in which the young drug abuser became hooked on heroin, but with recent tightening up of legislation in relation to drug prescribing by the medical profession, amphetamine has became more difficult to obtain and smoking cannabis has become more fashionable with teenagers. It is available as marijuana, made from dried leaves, or hashish, from the resin of the flowering tops. Colloquially, it is known as 'pot' or 'hash' and the hand-rolled cigarette in which this is smoked is known as a 'reefer' or a 'joint'. Both cannabis and hashish have a depressing effect on the central nervous system. They are usually smoked or inhaled and, taken in large doses, pleasant dreams and hallucinations may occur, so that cannabis is usually classified as an *hallucinogen*. However the hallucinogen which causes most serious problems amongst teenagers is the synthetic preparation L.S.D. (lysergic acid diethylamide) known colloquially as 'acid'. Hallucinogens appear to be particularly attractive to middle-class youth and to students. Cessation of the use of cannabis does not appear to cause any withdrawal symptoms and its position as a drug of dependence has been controversial. For many young people, cannabis parties are fashionable and cannabis has by now replaced pep pills. At such a party, a young person may be introduced to L.S.D. or hard drugs such as heroin or cocaine. More recently, mixtures of drugs have become fashionable. These are particularly dangerous, especially if an accidental overdose is administered, when it may be difficult to find out exactly what drugs have been incorporated in the mixture. Concern has also been expressed about drugs, particularly L.S.D., being slipped into a cup of coffee unknown to its imbiber.

At the back of all this is the pusher, who uses drug abuse to maintain a handsome living. There can be only one attitude towards his activities—outright condemnation.

SPECIFIC DRUGS

Alcohol

The increasing use of alcohol by young people is presenting a problem. The number of people under eighteen appearing in court charged with drunkenness has been rising in the last decade. Although serious addiction is rare before adult life, alcohol abuse remains a major problem in adolescence. As with other drugs, the role of accessibility is important. Shy, inhibited teenagers sometimes resort to alcohol in an attempt to bolster up their self-confidence. A student, for example, may have several drinks before going to an all-important date with a girl-friend, unaware that, should the situation arise, his sexual prowess is likely to be diminished. Alcohol depresses the central nervous system, but initially it produces relaxation and euphoria, although this is associated with impairment of judgment and poor co-ordination. The long-term results of over-indulgence in alcohol, for example, neuritis, cirrhosis (degeneration) of the liver and atrophy of the brain, may develop over the years with resulting serious physical and mental impairment and, ultimately, even death, in contradistinction to the earlier and more acute mortality associated with drug abuse.

Barbiturates (*see* also Chapter 18)
The abuse of barbiturates was traditionally confined to middle-age, especially in women who usually obtained their supply from a doctor's prescription, but in recent years young people have shown a tendency to obtain them illegally and abuse them. Adolescents are likely to take barbiturates in combination with another drug, for example, a cerebral stimulant such as amphetamine. Barbiturates are depressant to the central nervous system and the combination of a barbiturate with amphetamine ('purple hearts', 'French blues') seems to limit the unpleasant stimulant effect of amphetamine. Recently, the use of barbiturates by intravenous injection by adolescents has been causing concern.

Barbiturates are similar to alcohol in their effect. First there is the stage of disinhibition when the drug-taker exhibits excitement, irritability, talkativeness and trembling. Speech may become slurred and the individual is unsteady on his feet, the latter phenomenon being known as 'ataxia'. This stage is followed by drowsiness, confusion, and later coma if a large enough dose is consumed. The effects are of longer duration than alcohol. There are many derivatives of barbituric acid and the speed and duration of action of a particular member of this group depends on the chemical structure, preparations with longer chemical side-chains being destroyed more rapidly, thus having a shorter action.

Other sedative substances may be abused, for example, the

sleeping drug methaqualone (Mandrax), often with similar effects and side-effects of barbituates, but sometimes producing their own unpleasant and even dangerous sequelae.

Opiates

This group includes the natural derivatives of opium and also synthetic substances with a morphine-like effect, and includes opium, morphine, heroin, pethidine and methadone (physeptone).

Until 1959, people dependent on this group of drugs usually became addicted during the course of medical treatment. None of these individuals was under twenty-five years of age, and the majority were over fifty. By the end of the 1960s, there had been a vast increase in the number of opium addicts, and over half were under the age of twenty-five and almost a quarter under twenty. Amongst teenagers, heroin is the opiate of choice. Its duration of action is short (about two hours) but it produces an almost immediate feeling of well-being ('high' or 'buzz') during which the drug-taker feels happy and excited. In some persons, the imagination appears to be more vivid and they feel more intelligent. The effects of heroin wear off rapidly and, by the end of four hours, withdrawal symptoms are being experienced. Many of those dependent on drugs are apprehensive about withdrawal symptoms and a user may utilise this apprehension to obtain a 'fix' from a sympathetic doctor. The common withdrawal symptoms are, irritability, anxiety, yawning, running eyes and nose, restlessness, vomiting, diarrhoea, abdominal cramp and limb pains. Withdrawal symptoms seem to be most severe over the first two to three days after the cessation of the drug. If these withdrawal symptoms are severe, then the administration of a substitute narcotic drug, methadone, may be used under strict medical supervision. Recently, some anxiety has been expressed about the wisdom of this course as methadone itself gives rise to drug dependence, though less severe.

The euphoric effect is the property which predominantly produces dependence on heroin. Once dependent, the individual will neglect food and hygiene in a quest for heroin and it is this which contributes to the high death-rate—the addict saving money to buy his fix. Having obtained it, he may be so anxious to use it that he omits sterile precautions when injecting himself and so develops skin infections, or more seriously septicaemia (infection of the blood stream). The strength of heroin bought illegally may not be known, so that, inadvertently, the addict may take an overdose. This is particularly likely to occur since the introduction into this country of so-called Chinese heroin.

Although heroin is the opiate of choice, it is not easily available, so other opiates may be substituted. Morphine itself has been used, but is less potent in creating a state of euphoria, although otherwise its effect is very similar to that of heroin. Methadone (physeptone) is a synthetic analgesic. Its original introduction was greeted with enthusiasm, as it was thought that it did not produce dependence, but unhappily it is now known to do so. Its effects are similar to those of morphine and heroin, but are less dramatic. As mentioned above, its recent use at some drug treatment centres in an attempt to prevent withdrawal symptoms during treatment of other forms of opium addiction, is now having to be viewed with caution.

Cocaine

As it was common to combine barbiturates with amphetamines, so there was a period when it was relatively common to combine cocaine with heroin. Cocaine itself has a rapid effect, but it is not a narcotic and it is thought to counteract the narcotic effect of opiates when they are taken in combination. It is commonly sniffed, but teenagers also inject it intravenously. Cocaine is a cerebral stimulant, which increases intellectual function. Decisions are made rapidly and self-confidence is enhanced and it is these euphoriant effects which make cocaine so popular with the younger age group. Formerly, its use in medicine was as a local anaesthetic, but better local anaesthetic preparations are now available and it is now rarely used.

Amphetamine

Formerly amphetamine was valued for its stimulant effect on the central nervous system, causing a feeling of well-being almost amounting to exaltation, the subject being aware of increased mental activity and fatigue dropping away. It was introduced in the treatment of depression in the 1930s and also used as an appetite-suppressant in those who were overweight. The medical profession gradually became aware that patients could become habituated to its use, although abuse of amphetamine did not become a major problem until the 1960s when, as described previously, it was used by teenagers to enhance their enjoyment at the end of the day. With prolonged abuse of amphetamines, hallucinations and paranoid psychosis have been described and in some cases these have proved very difficult to treat.

Hallucinogens
This group of drugs is so called because one of their main effects is to produce hallucinations.

Cannabis
Cannabis belongs to this group of drugs, but in fact is a very mild hallucinogen, as are nutmeg and Morning Glory. Cannabis may be smoked or eaten, the effect of a smoke lasting for several hours. A smoker may feel 'high' and may become mildly disinhibited with an increasing sense of self-confidence. At teenage cannabis parties, teenagers may not progress beyond this stage, but with continued smoking, judgment regarding space and time become impaired and psychotic disturbances have been reported, such as thought-disorder, delusions and hallucinatory experiences. Perhaps the most unfortunate feature of cannabis smoking is the apathy which may be associated with it. The question of minimal brain damage caused by prolonged smoking of cannabis has been raised recently, but the matter is still *sub judice* and many people feel that the work on which the suggestion was based is suspect.

L.S.D.
The more potent hallucinogens include the synthetic preparation L.S.D. (lysergic acid diethylamide) D.M.T. (dimethyltriptamine), and D.E.T. (diethyltriptamine). Of these, the most commonly used is L.S.D. There is considerable evidence that the effects of these drugs and their residual action are closely allied to the individual's emotional state at the time of consuming the drug. Shortly after taking it, he develops feelings of detachment and may become visually hallucinated. Sometimes, in this state, he will behave dangerously, for example walking out of a window in a multi-storey block of flats in the belief that he can fly. Many drug-taking teenagers are aware of the risks and often a member of the group remains drug-free to act as a 'guard' for his fellows.

THE DRUG-TAKER

Classically, the drug-taker has been considered to have a dependent type of personality, even bordering on inadequacy, and needing a prop to bolster up his self-esteem. Many drugs will do just this, at least in the short term, and the resulting boost to self-confidence which the drug-taker obtains from an isolated dose encourages him to experiment, to take repeated doses and gradually to increase the amount of the drug as he becomes habituated, so that a pattern of drug-dependence develops, compensating for defects in his personality. So, if a drug-taker with this background accepts treatment and the drug is withdrawn, he is still left with his serious personality problems. Those treating him must be aware of this and the enormous amount of support which he will require as a substitute for the drug.

Apart from the problems of the individual, there have been major changes in our society in the post-war period. An older generation which grew up in a strong Christian tradition learned to work for rewards in the next world (as well as in this) and so were prepared to tolerate some degree of discomfort in the present but, since the Second World War, we have 'never had it so good' so perhaps it is not surprising that today's teenagers are looking for the pleasures of the moment.

Before the 1944 Education Act, when the brighter pupils were creamed-off for selective education, workers might see the bright young chap rise from the shop floor to management and might sometimes feel, however unrealistically, that perhaps their own conditions might improve. This is much less likely to happen nowadays, when ability is recognised early in life and opportunities for further education are available. There has been an increase in the complexity of life and many perceptive teenagers may sometimes be overwhelmed by the demands which society makes on them. With mechanisation in industry, there has been some decrease in job-satisfaction and many teenagers leaving school worry that the type of work they obtain on first entering employment will be that which they may have to do for the next forty to fifty years. If community leisure resources do not provide stimulation, these young people may become bored. Many teenagers have difficulty in appreciating what is renown and what is notoriety, and since in large educational establishments and factories they can feel depersonalised, they may be driven to seek the limelight. Many do this in a way which is acceptable to society, but for a proportion the glamour of drug-taking fills the vacuum. They initially start for the 'kick', but then they become hooked and find it difficult to refuse the drug, even if they wish to do so.

In the past, the not-so-bright son of a well-to-do family could have a position bought for him in society, so that he would be able to maintain the standard of living in which he had been brought up. Increasingly, academic qualifications are demanded and some of the duller off-spring of wealthy parents realise that, once they have to survive by their own efforts, their standard of living may drop dramatically. For such individuals drug-taking may provide a way out.

For some students, the change from a relatively structured, safe environment to an unsupervised life on the university or college campus may prove difficult and their longed-for freedom proves overwhelming. They may react to lack of support and feelings of loneliness by involvement in a group-culture that may include drug-taking.

So, although the classical 'inadequate personality' pattern may still underlie many cases of drug-abuse, we can see that there may be many causative factors for, and pathways to, dependence.

TREATMENT AND MANAGEMENT

In this country, a committee on drug abuse under the chairmanship of Lord Brain reported in 1961 and again in 1965. This committee took the view that the individual dependent on drugs should be regarded as suffering from mental disorder rather than exhibiting criminal behaviour and they compared drug addiction with an infectious illness. Just as certain sanctions were placed on individuals who suffered serious infectious diseases such as tuberculosis or typhoid, for the benefit of themselves and the community, and certain administrative demands were made on doctors, so a similar pattern of management was recommended for the treatment of the drug addict. The sick role of the drug-abuser continues to form the basis of treatment in this country at the present time and throughout the United Kingdom there are hospitals which have special units for the treatment of drug-takers. Legislation governing the prescription of habit-forming drugs has been tightened up and, in the case of the 'hard' drugs, only certain doctors are permitted to prescribe them. Nowadays, more stringent disciplinary procedures are taken against doctors abusing the regulations. In addition, the Home Office is notified of all registered addicts.

The early recognition of the problem of the drug-abuser appears to be important for the ultimate outcome and for this reason, teachers and other professional workers who may encounter drug-taking adolescents in the course of their work, have been the recipients of considerable propaganda and teaching efforts to try to enable them to recognise the early signs of drug misuse. This is particularly difficult, as adolescents experimenting on drugs will be at the stage when they are also experimenting with independence and are particularly unlikely to confide in their family or other key figures in their environment. There are many adolescents who are moody, irritable and aggressive, but in may be difficult to decide whether this is just a phase of adolescent development, or whether a drug-taking pattern has been introduced. However, suspicions may be aroused if a teenager has considerable difficulty in facing the day, comes home late at night, appears to have lost appetite and weight, and shows lack of normal inhibitions in conversation and behaviour.

Once the suspicion of drug-taking has arisen, there may be problems in persuading the teenager to seek medical advice. Occasionally, this can be done on general grounds and the family doctor may then be made aware of the family or teacher's suspicions. Tactful examination may reveal signs of needle marks at injection sites and analysis of blood and urine will confirm the presence of some drugs, though the detection of hallucinogens presents great difficulties. If the diagnosis is confirmed, involvement with a psychiatrist may be suggested, although again, it may be difficult to persuade the teenager to accept this advice. If he has become seriously mentally disturbed as a result of his drug-taking, admission to hospital under a section of the Mental Health Act 1959 may be required if he will not, or cannot, be co-operative.

Physical complications of drug-taking, particularly where 'mainlining' (intravenous injection) has been used, may require urgent attention, as serious infection can result. However, the treatment of urgent physical complications apart, the first aim of treatment is withdrawal from the drug on which the teenager has become dependent. This may be achieved in an out-patient setting, but in some instances, admission to hospital may be required. Where possible, this ought to be a unit specialising in the management of drug-addiction. Drug-abusers should *not* be admitted to a hospital ward for emotionally-disturbed adolescents, as these younsters are likely to glamourise the drug taker. The latter will be flattered by the attention which he receives and may even introduce other patients to the drug, whereas if he is in a special unit where all the other patients abuse drugs, he is unlikely to gain any special prestige from this addiction but may, in fact, benefit from being one of the first patients in the unit to give up his drug-taking. This will depend on the constructive therapeutic use of group pressures operating within the drug addiction unit.

Ideally, the drug of addiction is withdrawn, possibly under the cover of a major tranquilliser such as chlorpromazine or an hypnotic like chlormethiazole, but the danger here is of substitution of addiction to the hypnotic drug, in place of the drug to which the patient had originally became habituated. Therefore, this situation has to be closely monitored.

In the case of barbituate addiction, drug withdrawal must be in an in-patient setting because of the risk of convulsions in the withdrawal stage. Those addicts taking heroin intravenously are thought to be particularly attached to the 'needle habit' and, for this reason, it has been felt that the use of an oral opiate such as methadone at an intermediate stage in treatment would be beneficial. As mentioned earlier, there has been some re-thinking about this because one then has the problem of weaning the patient away from the methadone to which he is also likely to become dependent.

If the drug-abuse is being treated in an out-patient clinic and the dose of the drug involved is being reduced, it is essential that the prescriptions are given directly to the prescribing chemist, as otherwise the teenager may be tempted to alter the dose. Good communications between the clinic and the patient's family doctor are essential, as the patient is also likely to ask his family doctor for additional supplies of the drug. Other ruses may well be tried, such as approaching a strange general practitioner on the grounds of being a temporary resident.

Whilst the drug of addiction is being withdrawn, the adolescent must be helped to face up to his 'nakedness'. It is sometimes helpful to make him aware that he will be particularly vulnerable at this period and to aid him to find ways of support within his own environment. Many of these youngsters have what amounts to a 'social phobia'. They have marked difficulties in inter-personal relationships with their own and the opposite sex, their own generation and with adults. In extreme cases, they may find it difficult to eat in public places or shop on their own and a programme of social re-learning may have to be undertaken. In some therapeutic units, group therapy (*see* Chapter 19) is an adjunct to treatment, but at times the very thought of communicating in a group situation may drive these dependent teenagers away from the treatment setting. It is likely that, before coming for treatment, their main source of contact will have been within the drug-culture and obviously sustained contact with other drug-takers will make it difficult for the patient to withdraw from the drug for any length of time.

Working with young addicts places tremendous strain on the emotional resources of staff. It is extremely difficult to keep a balance between the needs of the patient and the view of society. It is all too easy to become over-identified with the drug-taker and condone minor infringements of the law. Therefore, essential features of all drug treatment centres are ongoing reviews of methods and constant attention to staff morale.

PROGNOSIS

It is still rather early to generalise about the outlook for those teenagers who have been taking drugs over the last decade, but follow-up studies are beginning to appear. Unhappily, a high mortality rate remains a consistent feature. In one London study, approximately one-fifth of those addicted to opiates were dead within five years, and of those surviving, about a third were off narcotics but a half were still involved.

In more general terms, it is postulated that drug-abuse is part of the 'uniform' adopted by a given generation of teenagers: it is to be hoped that, as the next generation arrives, they will adopt a safer and healthier means of working-through their problems. Meantime, we cannot afford to be facile in our expectations. We may show every sympathy to the individual teenager who has been caught in the toils of the drug habit, but we should deprecate the non-therapeutic use of drugs and do everything constructive that we can to eliminate the trend.

REFERENCES AND FURTHER READING

Bewley, T. H. 'An Introduction to Drug Dependence.' Brit. Journal. Hospital Medicine, 1970, *4*, 150.

Boyd, P. 'Drug Abuse and Addiction.' Ch. XIII in *Modern Perspectives in Adolescent Psychiatry*. Ed. J. Howells. Oliver & Boyd, 1971.

Chapple, P. A. L., Somekh, P. E., and Taylor, M. E. 'Follow-up of cases of Opium Addiction from the time of notification to the Home Office.' Brit. Med. J., 1972, *2*, 680.

D.H.S.S. *Medical Memorandum on Drug Dependence*. H.M.S.O., 1972.

H.M.S.O. *First inter-departmental report on drug abuse*. 1961.

H.M.S.O. *Drug Addiction. Second report interdepartmental committee*. 1965.

Scott, P. D. and Willcox, D. R. C. 'Delinquency and the Amphetamines.' Brit. J. Psychiat., 1965, *111*, 865.

Wilson, C. W. M. (Ed.). *Adolescent Drug Dependence*. Pergamon Press, 1968.

Wootton of Abinger. *Cannabis*. Report by the Advisory Committee on Drug Dependence. H.M.S.O., 1968.

World Health Organisation. *Expert Committee on Addiction-Producing Drugs*. 15th Report. W.H.O. Tech. P. Ser. 273, 1964.

*Young, J. *The Drugtaker*. Paladin, 1971.

* *Recommended selected reading.*

9 Developmental disorders

In the first chapter, the genetic and intra-uterine aspects of the development of the unborn child were discussed and reference was made to parental aspirations. As the new-born child develops, parental attitudes towards the infant become increasingly important and the parents' pride in his early achievements, or their distress at his discomfort, are normal emotions. Inevitably, they are concerned about his physical development, his weight gain, his stature, and his developmental accomplishments. The major developmental milestones recognised are:

Sitting without support	7 to 9 months
Standing with support	9 months
Walking	13 to 18 months
Feeding himself	15 to 18 months
Speech—one word with meaning	21 to 24 months
Combining two, three words and increasingly fluent	Two years
Bladder-sphincter control by day	$2\frac{1}{2}$ to 3 years
Bladder sphincter control by night	3 to 4 years
Anal-sphincter control	2 years

These skills are usually acquired by girls at a younger age than boys. Parents of a first child have no standard of comparison and if the first child, a girl, is followed by a son, parents may be concerned that there is a developmental delay and require reassurance.

Once a child acquires a skill, by and large it is for life, unless illness, for example meningitis, should intervene.

By adolescence, failure to gain developmental milestones should have been investigated and appropriate management instituted, but occasionally such investigation may have been omitted. With the onset of adolescence, the teenager may himself urge his parents to obtain help for him. Developmental problems presenting to the adolescent psychiatrist are, usually, stuttering (stammering), enuresis (bed-wetting) and encopresis (soiling).

Some of the developmental tasks of childhood are complex. For example, going to the toilet involves sufficient motor skills to cope with taking down pants, etc. Just as a child cannot learn to walk until certain tracts of the spinal cord mature (become myelinised) so it seems likely that maturation of other parts of the central nervous system may be necessary before other skills can be acquired. The question of *critical periods of learning* is also thought to be a factor. This will be referred to in the discussion of enuresis.

Speech demands a high degree of integration within the central nervous system. As an example, it is first necessary to assure oneself that the individual has the *capacity to learn to speak*. A child who is severely mentally-handicapped, or a very deaf child, will not learn as easily as one without a handicap, if he learns at all. Given then that the child has the capacity to learn to speak, the language he uses is environmentally determined. For example, if he is brought up in France he will probably speak French, but if in India, Gujurati, Punjabi or Hindustani may be his native language. Even if he learns English, he may speak with an Australian or American accent and within our island there is a great variety of accents and dialects. Sometimes interference with the process of learning may occur and speech that has been normally acquired may subsequently be lost, as in an adult who has had a cerebrovascular accident (a stroke), or who has sustained a head injury damaging a particular part of the brain. So, when competence in speech is used to assess children who present with developmental disorders, it is necessary to look at their capacity to learn, the learning environment and factors which may interfere with the learning process. It is now proposed to look at specific developmental problems presenting at an adolescent psychiatric clinic.

STUTTERING

As the child acquires speech, he may find it difficult to produce words as rapidly as he is thinking, he may hesitate as he has difficulty in finding the right word, or he may become 'hung up' on certain syllables so that a stutter results. Some people have talked of a physiological stutter or stammer associated with this age period, since a slight degree of impediment—usually temporary—is so common. Other children first develop a stutter when they start school and a very few may acquire it when they reach puberty. There appears to be a genetic factor associated with stuttering, in that some stutterers have a history of relatives with a similar difficulty. As with other developmental disorders, boys appear to be affected twice as frequently as girls. The maximum prevalence of stuttering is at the time that the children are learning to speak and there is a gradual decline, only about 1 per cent of children becoming persistant stutterers (Andrews and Harris, 1964).

At one period, it used to be thought that stuttering was associated with left-handedness and that incomplete cerebral dominance might be a factor in its causation. There was a time when children who were naturally left-handed were forced at school to become right-handed but, despite the above theory, Andrews and Harris found that there was no relationship between stuttering and left-handedness or change of handedness. Analysing findings obtained by examination of eighty stutterers surveyed during their last two years at primary schools, these authors found that stuttering tended to occur when a child appeared something of a misfit, having difficulties with social learning and intellectual functioning. Such children appeared to come from insecure homes, their mothers also giving a history of poor record at school and at work. On the other hand, stuttering associated with over-activity and irritability was suggestive of minimal cerebral dysfunction. Anxious children, whose parents have excessively high expectations of them may also become stutterers. Some studies have suggested that stutterers have an excess of emotional problems, but whether these are primary, or secondary to the emotional atmosphere and anxiety caused by the stutter, has yet to be ascertained. Contrariwise, Andrews and Harris found no association between the stutter and emotional disturbances.

In order to reduce the risk of emotional disturbance arising secondarily to the stutter, it is important that treatment of early stutters should be instituted by the age of four. Ideally, the child should have help before he has to face the stresses of the classroom. As in other developmental disorders, the medical role is to look at the child's capacity to speak fluently, to ascertain if intellectual retardation is present, or whether there may be other evidence of cerebral dysfunction. Deafness should also be excluded. If any physical defects are found these should be dealt with appropriately.

The learning environment may also be important and reduction of anxieties for the child and his family may be necessary. A specific attack on the symptom is usually made by the speech therapist. Various approaches are employed but one method is that described by Andrews and Harris as 'syllable stressed speech'. In this the child is taught to emphasise every syllable, giving time to each one so that the usual stresses are removed. Sometimes a metronome may be used to encourage the child in this (*see* also Chapter 19).

ENCOPRESIS (Soiling)

Encopresis, or soiling, occurs when a child fails to gain normal bowel control or, having gained control, later loses it. Most children are toilet-trained by two years of age, but the mentally retarded child may be considerably delayed in gaining control. Local physical disease of the bowel may also result in delayed anal-sphincter control; for example, a child who has severe constipation in infancy may have an anal fissure which is a particularly painful tear of the skin around the anus (back passage). Hirschprung's disease, in which a disorder of the nerve cells in the bowel causes megacolon or dilatation of the large bowel, and is also associated with constipation. In some cases of severe constipation, loose motions may pile up behind the hard stool and may leak through the anus, giving a false impression of diarrhoea. These conditions

may result in a child appearing to lose control of evacuation and he
may then present with soiling.

The learning environment is also important. It has been observed
that in some homes there is little encouragement for the child to
become toilet trained, so there may be encopresis and associated
enuresis (urinary incontinence). These children are often quite un-
ashamed of their incontinence. The opposite extreme is the home
where the mother has emotional over-concern about toilet training
and here there may be considerable conflict between what Anthony
has called 'the potting couple', that is the mother and the child.
Bowel evacuation becomes a battle-ground, where ultimately the
child is victorious. In this latter situation, the history is usually of
early achievement of bowel control with soiling recurring, particularly about the time the child starts school. In other instances,
encopresis may appear in response to specific stresses, particularly
in the home environment. These children are often continent when
in hospital, only to relapse upon return to the problems of the outside world.

In the Isle of Wight study, 1·3 per cent of the boys and 0·3 per
cent of the girls were reported to be soiling at least once a month
and about half of these children were soiling at least once a week in
their last year of primary school. Again, the predominance of this
condition in boys is noted. The disorder tends to decline through
the years at primary school and rarely persists after puberty.

The Freudian view of personality development suggests that in
the initial stages of development the child gets its emotional
gratification through sucking at the mother's breast, or putting its
hands in its mouth. This is known as the oral stage. At the next
stage, it is suggested that gratification is largely centred on anal
sensation. Further development of Freud's theory suggests that
particular types of personality may be related to excessive fixation
of libido at an immature stage. The obsessional personality is said
to be especially associated with fixation at the anal phase of the
child's development. If this were actually so, one might anticipate
that encopretic children would subsequently have obsessional personalities or present with an obsessional neurosis (*see* Chapter 12).
There appears to be no evidence to support this and Dr. J. Ross,
examining children who presented with obsessional symptoms, did
not find a history of encopresis in any. Rather, the literature

suggests that these children who have developmental difficulties involving encopresis may present later with conduct disorders, particularly stealing.

Prevention is perhaps the first stage of management. The motto should always be 'placid, painless potting'. However, when soiling has occurred, it may be necessary to organise bowel evacuation by combined use of laxatives and enemas followed by intensive retraining of bowel habit. The use of modified-reward schedule, a form of behaviour therapy, may be particularly useful. Sometimes an initial period in hospital may be necessary. As with other developmental disorders, there may be secondary emotional problems for which help will be required, and the actual role of emotional disorders in relation to encopresis has yet to be established.

ENURESIS (Wetting)

Enuresis is the failure to develop normal bladder function (when it is known as primary enuresis) or the loss of bladder control previously gained (when it is known as secondary or onset enuresis). During the pre-school period, the majority of children gradually gain bladder control, usually becoming dry during the day sooner than at night. Persistent bed-wetting is known as nocturnal enuresis, and this is more common than diurnal enuresis although often the two are associated.

Approximately 12 per cent of children in this country still wet their beds at four years of age and in the Isle of Wight study, 4.3 per cent of boys wet their pants or beds at least once a month and over half of these were wet at least once per week. In contrast, 2.4 per cent of the girls wet their beds or pants at least once per month and 1.9 per cent were wet at least once a week. At puberty, the majority of boys and girls have become dry and it is suggested that less than one per cent of children continue to be wet after puberty. Again, as with other developmental disorders, the predominance in boys is noted and also the tendency to spontaneous remission with age in both sexes. These factors must always be considered when assessing the effect of therapeutic intervention. About one in eight enuretics are also encopretic. Although boys are more liable to bed-wetting, the number of boys and girls wetting during the day is approximately equal.

Again, the capacity to learn must be examined. It is recognised that in a minority of children bed-wetting may be associated with organic disease. Although their number is small, it is important that these are recognised. Organic factors include:

1. Urinary tract infection.
2. Obstruction of the lower urinary tract, which may give rise to urinary retention with overflow analogous to the spurious diarrhoea described under Encopresis.
3. Bladder paralysis which may be related to disease of the spinal cord, for example, children with spina bifida are now surviving as a result of surgical intervention and antibiotics and are often affected thus.
4. Occasionally a young child developing diabetes may present with incontinence due to a large quantity of urine being secreted as a result of the disease.
5. Congenital abnormality, such as displacement of one of the passages of the urinary tract. Wetting during the day as well as at night is particularly likely to be associated with organic pathology.

All children referred to a psychiatrist should have a physical examination as part of their initial assessment, and this is absolutely essential for the child presenting with enuresis. The urine should be examined in the laboratory for evidence of infection, or abnormal excretion of protein or sugar. Occasionally special investigations such as blood tests and X-rays may also be required, but this depends on the clinical judgment of the medical practitioner.

Incontinence of urine may occur in association with epileptic attacks and the child who wets his bed infrequently may have nocturnal epilepsy. In the primary school child, enuresis may occur as an isolated symptom but its association at times with other developmental disorders such as delay in speech development and bowel control, together with immature brainwave pattern as measured by the E.E.G. or electro-encephalogram (a brain wave test which examines the rhythmic electrical discharges from the brain), suggests that it may be part of an overall developmental immaturity. In enuretics presenting at an adolescent clinic, it is less likely to be an isolated symptom, particularly where there is urinary incontinence both day and night and children who present with conduct disorders often have a history of previous enuresis (*see* next Chapter). However, in the Isle of Wight study it was noticed that enuresis was associated equally with children who had neurotic and those who had anti-social symptoms.

It has been observed that nocturnal enuresis is commoner in the lower social classes and mention has also been made of parental attitudes to toilet training when discussing encopresis. Attention has been drawn to the number of enuretic children growing up in institutions and many enuretic children had an admission to hospital or other separation from home about the time they would have been expected to gain bladder-sphincter control. It has been suggested that there are critical periods of learning and that enuresis is the outcome of interference with toilet training at this vital age. Jealousy over the birth of a sibling has also been considered a factor in both enuresis and encopresis, the mechanism in operation here being one of regression.

In a proportion of cases, there is a family history of enuresis, particularly affecting males. This may reflect some hereditary disorder of maturation or, in some cases, may represent an aberrant form of upbringing.

The literature is full of almost sadistic methods of treatment going as far back as the Middle Ages and one has occasionally met the enuretic parent of an enuretic child who has declined to have the child subjected to the 'torture' which fell to the parental lot. The advent of the washing machine and the spin dryer may result in pressures on present-day enuretic children being lessened. The two keystones in rational treatment today are:

1. Drugs.
2. Behaviour therapy.

Drug treatment of enuresis

Fortuitously, during the treatment of depression with tricyclic antidepressant drugs, it was noted that some patients with enuresis became continent. As a result of this, Imipramine and other tricyclic anti-depressants have been used in the treatment of enuresis with considerable success. Before this beneficial side-effect of the tricyclic drugs was known, it was thought that the enuretic child slept too deeply and did not waken as the bladder pressure increased. To combat this, drugs of the amphetamine group were in vogue and it was thought that by lightening the level of sleep, bed-wetting would be less likely. However, with the abuse of amphetamine preparations, this particular drug is not recommended at the present time. The theory of its use has in fact altered and, rather than being used to alter the level of sleep, it has been thought that it might be of value in making conditioning easier. Formerly it was sometimes used in association with behaviour therapy methods.

Drugs acting through the parasympathetic nervous system on the smooth muscle of the bladder have been used in the past, such as tincture of belladonna and propantheline (Probanthine) but results have not been encouraging. Restricting fluid intake after 6.00 p.m. and lifting the child to pass urine at the parental bedtime have also been used but seem to be unhelpful in most cases.

Some children become dry when sleeping in a strange environment, for example on admission to hospital, but do not remain dry on returning home. This has various causes and it is important to explain about this to parents and children, as the former sometimes feel that this symptom is under conscious control and that bed-wetting at home is an aggressive act. It is in this way that secondary emotional problems can arise.

Behaviour therapy or conditioning treatment (*see* also Chapter 19)
Today this involves the use of a buzzer and pad. The pad consists of two wire mats which are placed on top of a water-proof sheet covering the mattress, a draw-sheet being used to separate the wire mats from each other. Then the usual sheet is placed firmly on top and tucked in well to hold the mats in position. A lead from the mat is attached to the alarm (bell or buzzer). When bed-wetting occurs the urine passed acts as an electrolytic solution and the electric circuit is completed, causing the current to be conducted from the wire mats, which act as electrodes, to the buzzer, which makes a loud noise and wakes the patient. With adequate supervision, this form of treatment is probably the method of choice and has a high success rate. It is important that the teenager and his family are ful-

ly informed about making up the bed correctly with the wire mats. Ideally, the draw-sheet between the two wire mats should be flannelette and if a thin draw-sheet is used it may have to be doubled.

Used properly, the buzzer and pad is not dangerous but occasionally buzzer ulcers occur through inadequate instruction. This is particularly likely to occur if the battery has run down, if the buzzer fails to waken the patient, or if such a small quantity of urine is passed on to the bed that it fails to set off the alarm.

The child is encouraged to sleep naked from the waist down. When the buzzer sounds as the electrical circuit is completed, he should waken and then switch off the alarm, go to the toilet and finish the evacuation of his bladder. Following this the bed should be remade. The time which the alarm takes to awaken him should be noted and it is useful to measure the size of the patch of urine. As this is a battery-run system, the batteries will require renewing from time to time. It is always important to ensure that the system has been switched on when the child retires to bed and switched off on rising in the morning.

The buzzer should be used until the child has been dry for three or four successive weeks and should probably be kept in reserve for about six months in view of the high relapse rate. If a cure is not achieved within four months, it is unlikely that improvement with this method of treatment will result. Occasionally young children may not awaken with the conventional buzzer and amplification may be required.

SPECIFIC LEARNING DISORDERS

When he is introduced to compulsory education, the developing child is expected to acquire a further range of complex skills including reading, writing, spelling and arithmetic. Some children who are mentally handicapped have difficulty in acquiring all of these but other children have a particular difficulty with one modality. Difficulty in reading is sometimes termed 'dyslexia', difficulty with writing 'dysgraphia', and difficulty with figures 'dyscalculia'. Even when due allowance is made for intellectual handicap, some children continue to have quite specific difficulties with one of the three Rs. Although arithmetical difficulty may cause distress to the child, it is less of a social handicap than difficulty in learning to read. Even in adolescence, although patients rarely present to a psychiatrist with a reading difficulty as their sole problem, this may be an important feature in the total situation. Apart from specific learning problems, factors in the adolescent's capacity to learn, relating to difficulties with hearing or marked spasticity, should be identified and appropriate measures instituted. Any other disease processes or social disadvantages interfering with learning should also have been diagnosed and dealt with. It is known that the learning environment is important in the acquisition of reading skills and that children from large families may have particular difficulty in acquiring skills if parental expectations with regard to education are low. Some children with a reading difficulty have a positive family history, in that one or other of the parents had similar problems and it has been postulated that there may be a genetic element in this. On the other hand, the parent who had difficulty himself in learning to read may be over-sympathetic towards his child in a similar situation and may make few demands on him to learn to read.

In the Isle of Wight study, 'reading backwardness' was defined by Rutter and his colleagues as a reading age of twenty-eight months or more below the chronological age, when tested on accuracy or comprehension measures, and they included children with a low level of intelligence. It was found that 6·6 per cent of all the children had a general reading backwardness. The term, 'Reading Retardation' was used to describe children who were *seriously* handicapped in reading, where allowance was made for their general intellectual abilities. The prevalence rate for reading retardation was 3·7 per cent.

Unfortunately, most of the children with reading difficulties had received no special help in reading and when re-examined after two years had made little headway. It was noted that boys were more likely to have reading retardation than girls and this was associated with a history of delay in speech and language development. Rutter stated that specific reading retardation could be included amongst the group of developmental disorders of childhood. It has sometimes been called 'Specific Developmental Dyslexia' and has been regarded as a particularly severe condition, resistant to remedial teaching. The learning difficulty is confined to reading and spelling and it may be due essentially to a *visuo-spatial* abnormality, characterised by slowness in word recognition and an inability to discriminate between words of similar visual form; there is often reversal of letters, transposition of letters or *audiophonic* abnormalities where there is an inadequate auditory discrimination of speech sounds. Occasionally, both difficulties may be present simultaneously, when a particularly severe dyslexia results.

Some children with reading difficulties may have other evidence of delay in development, for example clumsiness and poor right–left discrimination. Identification of children with reading backwardness is essential, and obviously the earlier this can be done the better. Many children progressing from primary to secondary school continue to have marked reading difficulties and, as the Advisory Committee on Handicapped Children recommended to the Department of Education and Science, remedial help should be available to all children, including those who are backward in reading and those with reading retardation. Use of oral learning methods is important for these children, and there is no doubt that they require extra staff time. The problem should not be seen as one of very young children only: the Advisory Committee on Handicapped Children specifically mentions action at secondary school level, partly as a continuation of help for backward readers diagnosed at an earlier stage and partly to pick up those unfortunates whose disorder may have gone unnoticed before.

TICS

Tics or habit spasms are involuntary movements of muscles or groups of muscles. To the observer they may initially appear to serve some purpose, for example, eye blinking, but it soon becomes apparent that the movements are purposeless. The upper part of the body is most commonly affected, particularly the face. In more severe cases, there is extension downwards, with involvement of the whole head, neck or shoulders and in the most severely affected the trunk and limbs as well. Isolated phenomena such as sniffing, grunting or other vocal tics, may occasionally occur separately, but more commonly are associated with involvement of other muscle groups.

Size of the problem

It has been estimated that approximately 5 per cent of children have a history of tics occurring before the age of seven. Several studies have shown that tics occur more commonly in boys than in girls, three to four boys being affected for every girl but, in contrast, in the Isle of Wight study, the three children found to have *frequent* tics were all girls.

Corbett and his colleagues in a study of tiqueurs (*i.e.*, individuals with tics) presenting to a psychiatric hospital (both child and adult psychiatric departments) and at a child guidance clinic, found that the mean age at first attendance was 7·3 years and only one-fifth of the sample of a hundred and eighty patients presented for the first time in adolescence. In their study it was noted that tics never occurred in isolation and, by comparison with a total patient population, the tiqueurs tended to have an increased frequency of speech disorders, encopresis, and obsessional and hypochodriacal symptoms, but *less* evidence of conduct disorder than in the total disturbed child patient sample. They found a family history of tics in 10 per cent of their tiqueurs.

Although tics are here classified under developmental disorders, the cause of the symptoms has yet to be established. Many tiqueurs are referred to paediatric departments, suggesting that some workers feel that there may be an organic background. This appeared to be supported by Professor Pasamanick's demonstration that there had been a higher proportion of pregnancy complications in the mother of tiqueurs as compared with a matched control group. More recent work, however, has failed to confirm a Pasamanick's findings.

The increased association of tics with the male sex, the age of onset of the symptom and its improvement with increasing age, has encouraged some workers to regard tics as a developmental disorder and in the provisional classification of child psychiatric disorder for the International Classification of Disease (9th revision) tics were included under developmental disorders.* However, the majority of development disorders were associated with conduct disorder and the evidence from Corbett's study (above) and the fact that, on follow-up, many of the tiqueurs proved to have emotional

* When the 9th revision was published tics were not classified as a developmental disorder.

symptoms with anxiety predominating would indicate that it is premature to regard tics simply as a developmental disorder.

The referral of tiqueurs to a child or adolescent psychiatrist suggests that emotional factors are considered to be important. In no study has there been good evidence of acute emotional precipitants, but there is no doubt that many tiqueurs are greatly embarrassed by their symptoms, so undoubtedly secondary emotional factors may arise. A further theory put forward has been that tics are conditioned avoidance-responses, initially evoked by distress and reinforced by the subsequent reduction in anxiety. As a consequence of this, treatment by learning-theory methods (*see* Chapter 19) has been attempted.

At the time of writing, haloperidol (*see* Chapter 18) one of the butyrophenone group of drugs, is probably the most commonly used method of treatment. It is not curative, but may produce marked alleviation of the movements, to the sufferer's great relief. *Gilles de la Tourette* Syndrome was described by a physician of that name in 1885. It has also been called the 'Convulsive Tic Syndrome'. It consists of multiple motor tics with vocal utterances which are usually obscenities (coprolalia). It is likely that this syndrome is a particularly severe form of tic and not an entity in itself. It is very distressing for patient and relatives alike and, until haloperidol became available, proved very resistant to treatment. Nowadays some degree of relief is possible in many of the cases—fortunately the condition is relatively rare.

THE HYPERKINETIC SYNDROME

As with tics, there is considerable doubt as to how this syndrome should be classified. It is included in this Chapter on developmental disorders, but whilst many children presenting with this syndrome have associated organic brain pathology this is not always the case. As with tics, an international study group examining those diagnostic entities which might be included in the ninth revision of the International Classification of Disease under the heading of 'Child psychiatric disorders', decided there was a need for a subcategory entitled Hyperkinetic Disorders. For the time being, in the absence of further evidence this should be listed under developmental disorder (when the 9th revision was published this syndrome was in a category of its own).

As with other developmental disorders, the hyperkinetic syndrome is more common in boys than in girls. The syndrome becomes less severe with increasing age, to the extent that in adolescence many formerly over-active patients become under-active so that the hyperkinetic syndrome is not a major problem in adolescence. In the Isle of Wight survey, only one child was considered to have the hyperkinetic syndrom in the population of two thousand 9 to 11 year olds. As increasing numbers of child psychiatrists become available and as their training improves, one would anticipate that the majority of hyperkinetic children will have been screened and recognised at least during primary school stage. If so, the numbers presenting undiagnosed to those working with adolescents should decrease.

The clinical history is that of a child who, soon after he learns to walk, becomes the bane of his mother's life on account of his over-activity, distractibility and short attention span, punctuated by aggressive outbursts, the last often being provoked by the most trivial frustration. Many of these hyperkinetic children present superficially with cheerful, endearing features, but their lack of normal social inhibitions is marked. They have considerable difficulty in learning socially required behaviour such as, for example, road sense and so they require more than average supervision. Dr. Ounstead has coined the term 'hyperpaedophiliac' to describe the parental response to the excessive demands which are placed upon them.

Less severely over-active children may not be seen as a problem by their parents, who merely regard them as unduly lively and boisterous, but they may become a problem on entering school, when they find it difficult to sit still in the classroom and the teacher finds their distractibility and low tolerance of frustration too demanding. All hyperkinetic children merit a full assessment and investigation so that underlying factors, such as some organic disorder may be detected. The management consists of helping the parents and the school to work out a routine for the child, the simple use of behaviour therapy methods and, in some instances, drugs. Amphetamine used to be the drug of choice, but in view of the recent abuse of this drug, it has fallen out of favour and the phenothiazines and butyrophenones (*see* Chapter 18) have been used instead.

REFERENCES AND FURTHER READING

Illingworth, R. F. *The Normal Child.* J. A. Churchill, London. 4th Edtn., 1968.

Stuttering

Andrews, K. and Harris, M. *The Syndrome of Stuttering.* Clinics in Developmental Medicine No. 17. Heinemann, London, 1964.
Ingram, T. T. F. 'Disorders of Speech in Childhood.' Brit. J. Hosp. Medicine, 1969, *2*, 1608.

Encopresis

Bellman, M. 'Studies in Encopresis.' Acta. Paed. Scan., 1966, Suppl. 170.
Berg, I. and Jones, K. V. 'Functional Faecal Incontinence in Children.' Arch. Dis. Child., 1964, *39*, 465.
MacGregor, M. 'Chronic Constipation in Children in *Psychosomatic Aspects of Paediatrics.* Ed. R. McKeith and J. Sandler, Pergamon Press, 1961.

Enuresis

Editorial. 'Causes of Enuresis.' Brit. Med. J., 1969, *1*, 63.
Forsythe, W. I. and Redman, A. 'Enuresis and The Electric Alarm—200 Cases.' Brit. Med. J., 1970, *1*, 211.
Kolvin, I., McKeith, R. and Meadow, R. (Eds.) *Recent Advances in Bladder Control and Enuresis.* Heinemann, 1973.
Werry, J. 'Emotional Factors in Enuresis Nocturnal.' Develop. Med. Child. Neurol., 1965, *7*, 563.
Young, G. 'The Problem of Enuresis.' Brit. J. Hosp. Medicine, 1969, *2*, 628.

Reading difficulties

Department of Education and Science. *Children with Specific Reading Difficulties.* Report of Advisory Committee on Handicapped Children. H.M.S.O., 1972.
Mason, A. W. 'Specific (Developmental) Dyslexia.' Develop. Med. Child Neurol., 1967, *9*, 183.
Rutter, M. 'The Concept of "Dyslexia"' in 'Planning for better learning.' Clinics in Developmental Med., Ed. Wolff, P. U. and McKeith R., 1969, No. 33. Heinemann.

Tics

Connell, P. H., Corbett, J. A., Horne, B. J., and Mathews, A. M. 'Drug treatment of adolescent tiqueurs.' Brit. J. Psychiat., 1967, *113*, 375.

Corbett, J. A., Mathews, A. M., Connell, P. H. and Shapiro, D. A. 'Tics and Gilles de la Tourettes Syndrome: A follow-up study and critical review.' Brit. J. Psychiat., 1969, *115*, 1229.

Fernando, S. J. M. 'Gilles de la Tourette Syndrome: A Report on 4 Cases and a review of published case reports.' Brit. J. Psychiat., 1967. *113*, 607.

Kelman, D. H. 'Gilles de la Tourette Disease in Children: A review of the literature.' J. Child Psychol. Psychiat., 1965, *6*, 219.

Pasamanick, B. and Kawi, A. 'A study of the association of pre-natal and para-natal factors with the development of tic in children.' J. Paediat., 1956, *48*, 596.

Rutter, M., Tizard, J. and Whitmore, K. *Education, Health & Behaviour.* Longman, 1970.

Rutter, M., Lebovici, S., Eisenberg, L., Smeznevsky, A. V., Sadoun, R., Brooke, E. and Lin Psung Yi. 'A Tri-axial classification of Mental Disorders in Childhood. An International Study.' J. Child Psychol. and Psychiat., 1969, *10*, 41.

Torup, E. 'A Follow-up study of Children with Tics.' Act Paediat., 1962, *51*, 261.

Hyperkinetic syndrome

Editorial. 'Hyperactivity in Children.' Brit. Med. Journal, 1975, *4*, 123.

Eisenberg, B. G. L. 'Psychiatric Implications of Brain Damage in Children.' Psychiat. Quart., 1957, *31*, 72.

Ingram, T. T. S. 'A Characteristic Form of Over-active Behaviour in Brain-damaged Children.' J. Ment. Sci., 1956, 102, *550*, 558.

Ounstead, C. 'The Hyperkinetic Syndrome in Epileptic Children.' Lancet, 1955, *2*, 303.

Rutter, M. L., Shaffer, D. and Sturge, C. (prepared by). *A Guide & Multi-axial Classification Scheme for Psychiatric Disorders in Childhood and Adolesence.* Institute of Psychiatry. London.

Solomons, G. 'Child Hyper-activity: Diagnosis, Treatment.' Texas Medicine, 1967, *63*, 52.

Stewart, M. A., Pitts, F. N. Jnr., Craig, A. G. and Dieres, F. W. 'The Hyperactive Child Syndrome.' Am. J. Orthopsych., 1966, *36*, 861.

10 Conduct disorders and juvenile delinquency

To the psychiatrist, conduct disorder or anti-social disorder refers to a pattern of behaviour giving rise to social disapproval and which is not part of any other psychiatric condition, such as psychosis or personality disorder.

Delinquency is a legal concept and juvenile delinquents are those young people appearing before juvenile courts who are convicted of indictable (serious) offences. By definition, juveniles are aged 10 to 17 years. Obviously a change in the law can alter the number of offenders; for example, attempted suicide in England could result in prosecution until the passage of the Suicide Act in the last decade, one result of which was that attempted suicide was no longer an offence. As ten is the age of criminal responsibility, a child cannot be charged with an offence below this age. A child under ten whose anti-social behaviour is causing great concern may be committed to the care of the local authority if he is regarded as being beyond parental control.

Illegal behaviour has a narrower connotation than behaviour giving rise to social disapproval. For example, lying, swearing, bullying and defiance fall definitely in the latter category but do not constitute delinquency. If conduct-disorder is not defined too strictly, then many children with problems of delinquent behaviour could also be diagnosed as having a conduct disorder. Some psychiatrists feel that the term 'conduct-disorder' should not include those delinquents who appear to have normal personality development but who live in a high delinquency area (*i.e.,* socio-cultural delinquency which will be discussed later).

Some conduct-disordered children have also been noted to have emotional problems and the term 'mixed conduct and neurotic disorder' has been used to describe this group. Further studies of such children suggest that those in the mixed conduct and neurotic disordered group have more in common with a pure conduct disorder, than with a pure neurotic-disorder group. As with developmental disorders, delinquency and conduct disorders are both more common in males than females. For example, in the Isle of Wight studies 34 boys and 9 girls were considered to have a pure conduct disorder when screened in their last year at primary school and in addition, there were 22 boys and 5 girls with mixed conduct and neurotic disorder, giving a total of 56 boys and 14 girls having features of conduct disorder. In their last year of secondary school on the Isle of Wight, 39 boys and 9 girls (2·1 per cent of the total age matched population) were found to have a conduct disorder and 29 boys and 16 girls (1·9 per cent of the total) were found to have a mixed conduct and neurotic disorder, *i.e.,* an overall total of 68 boys and 25 girls.

In a national survey of children born in the first week of March 1946 (Douglas *et al.*) it was found that 13·7 per cent of males had been convicted of indictable offences up to the age of 17. However, it must be remembered that, in addition, many juveniles are cautioned by the police and others are found guilty of non-indictable offences. Boys predominate over girls in most of the psychiatric studies of conduct disorder, the ratio tending to be of the order of 2 to 1 or 3 to 1, whereas about 7 to 8 boys are convicted on an indictable offence for every girl so convicted. These figures must be interpreted with caution. It has been noted that many more males are in adult prisons than women, whereas women predominate amongst psychiatric hospital patients. It is possible that society may take a tougher line with male than female offenders, but there is also evidence that the type of offence committed varies with sex. Boys are more likely to be charged with aggressive behaviour than girls, who more often come to attention as being in need of care and protection, the modern equivalent of 'in moral danger'. Youths 'on the run' may well steal, or take and drive a vehicle to further their escape plans, whereas girls are more likely to hitch a lift and perhaps become the victim of a sexual offence—the traditional active male and passive female roles again in evidence.

Some years ago, the sight of an individual appearing half-undressed in the street would have been regarded by the majority of people as a sign of serious insanity. Today with the occurrence of 'streaking', the diagnosis would be less certain, so that always when considering normalities and abnormalities of behaviour, the cultural environment must be taken into account.

CLINICAL FEATURES

These are self-explanatory. The young person or someone in his environment becomes concerned about his anti-social behaviour which may be tending to escalate. A mother may notice that her house-keeping money is rather less than she had expected it to be and her suspicions are aroused. Resulting from this, she keeps a careful check and is gradually aware that small amounts are being pilfered. Her next task is to identify the culprit and then, according to her degree of concern and sophistication, she may approach the family doctor, probation officer, social worker, head teacher or clergyman. Discussion at this stage with school staff may provoke a reaction of surprise since, as far as school is concerned, the culprit is a happy, conforming pupil. In other instances, parents may be concerned because of their child's inability to fit in with family standards. He may be untruthful, disobedient, cruel to the family pets, or may manifest aggressive behaviour towards his siblings. Alternatively, the anti-social behaviour may make its first appearance in the school setting, where a pupil or member of staff may report the absence of money or belongings and investigation reveals the culprit. According to the seriousness of the offence, the school after consultation with the parents may deal with the matter internally or the police may be brought in. Almost inevitably, however, law enforcing agencies become involved when offences are committed outside the home or school environment, as for example with shop-lifting.

Children or adolescents with a conduct disorder may display a range of behavioural patterns including lying, defiance, bullying, offences against property (shop-lifting, other forms of stealing, breaking and entering, taking and driving vehicles), offences against the person, ranging from an aggressive episode to grievous bodily harm, manslaughter or murder. Sexual offences may also be included but these are dealt with elsewhere. The list is a formidable and rather sobering one.

CLASSIFICATION

Classifications in medicine may be descriptive, aetiological, prognostic or therapeutic. Let us now consider conduct disorder under each of these headings.

In conduct disorder, *descriptive* classifications are dealt with by a description of the offence and of the offender. Traditionally, offences are categorised as (a) offences against the person and, (b) offences against property. Some offences have been examined in depth, particularly murder, taking and driving offences, and absconding. Noteworthy is Rich's examination of stealing. As a result of his examination of boys at a remand home who had been charged with theft he describes five sub-groups:

1. 'Marauding', in which a small group of boys undertake a theft somewhat impulsively.
2. 'Proving' offences, when a boy sets out to prove his prowess or virility to himself, almost as a form of reassurance. Offences in this category are usually solitary. Taking and driving offences are sometimes of this nature.
3. 'Comforting' offences. Often these are stealing from parents, or impulsive solitary offences, as a substitute for lack of affection.
4. 'Secondary' offences. These are often planned with a definite idea of what may be stolen.
5. Other offences: in this group were those who could not be classified in the other four categories.

It is surprising that individual offences have not been studied in more depth. If the pattern of stealing commences at a very early age with pilfering in the home environment, is this of more significance than where the first anti-social behaviour is manifest in adolescence? There is an urgent need for long term follow-up on specific behavioural problems in order to answer apparently simple questions like this.

There have been many attempts to provide descriptive classifications of offenders. For convenience these will be dealt with in the next section.

An aetiological (causative) classification Behaviour is seen as a learnt response. It seems appropriate to examine it under the headings already used when discussing developmental disorders namely, capacity to learn, interference with the learning process, and the learning environment.

Capacity to learn

In the last century, an Italian psychiatrist Dr. Cesare Lombroso, drew attention to the concept of 'the born criminal'. In Lombroso's view, many criminals had physical attributes suggestive of primitive man. Lombroso regarded their bestial behaviour as being related to a general constitutional inferiority. These views are not accepted today. Nevertheless, there now is a growing amount of evidence to suggest that the delinquent's pattern of behaviour may not be entirely under his own control. The following influences may adversely affect the capacity to learn.

Genetic factors

Dr. Peter Scott, reporting on a W.H.O. conference on problems of deviant social behaviour and delinquency refers to a paper by Dr. Mednick in which it was found that there was an association between criminality in fathers and sons. A sample of adopted children demonstrated an unexpected and strikingly significant association between criminality of the adoptee and of his biological father, much more than that between the adoptee and his adoptive father. Professor Lee Robins in her study *Deviant Children Grown-up* has noted that the offspring of alcoholic or socio-pathic fathers were likely to develop similar traits, even if the two generations had never been in contact. These two studies appear to refute the suggestion that it is purely the environment which such fathers provide for their developing offspring, rather than genetic influences, which contribute to the pattern of deviant behaviour.

Dr. D. J. West and his colleagues have been carrying out a longitudinal study on 400 boys resident in South London. These youths were first contacted at the age of 8 when in primary school and have been followed up over a 10-year period. One-fifth became officially delinquent and factors particularly distinguishing the delinquent group were the presence of parental criminality, low income and poor parental example. Dr. West comments that although the boys were not seen until at least 8 years of age, the family factors had already been present for a long time.

Chromosomes
With the help of the electron microscope we have learned to analyse normal and abnormal chromosome patterns as described in Chapter 1. One of the abnormalities recognised is the XYY syndrome, in which the male has an extra Y chromosome. At an early stage of research of this condition some of these individuals were found in a special security hospital and were noted to have particularly aggressive behaviour and to be exceptionally tall. Scott and Kahn, reporting on a case at a Cropwood conference, suggested that persons with this chromosomal picture tend to become the black sheep of otherwise respectable families and start their offences, which are usually against property rather than persons, some five years younger than a control group of males manifesting anti-social behaviour but who have a normal chromosomal pattern. Obviously, further work has to be done on this syndrome before a final evaluation can take place and follow-up studies on the Edinburgh new-born sample will be particularly important here.

Other factors
A few years ago Dr. Denis Williams described a restrospective review of electro-encephalograms performed on subjects in custody for crimes of aggression. Those who were regarded as habitually aggressive tended to have abnormal E.E.G.s when compared with individuals committed for violent crimes, but not regarded as habitually aggressive. The preponderance of abnormal E.E.G.s in the habitually-agressive group persisted, even after subjects who were mentally retarded, epileptic or had suffered from a major head injury were excluded. Dr. Williams's findings are in line with those of earlier studies.

The work of Stella Chess and her co-workers referred to in

Chapter 1 also suggests that personality traits are not solely the outcome of child-rearing practices. The importance of intelligence in relation to delinquency has been argued to and fro since it became possible to measure the trait. Sir Cyril Burt found that juvenile delinquents were intellectually dull, but this was later refuted by the work of other psychologists. Some workers considered that the contribution of intellectual limitation might well result in a higher rate of *detection* of delinquency rather than being a contributory factor to the actual delinquency. However, in the most recent study by West, lower intelligence does appear to be a major predictive factor in delinquency.

Interference with the learning process
In Chapter 1, Pasamanick's theory of the continuum of reproductive casualty was referred to, suggesting that at conception the future individual was as nearly perfect as that person could be, but that various insults in the intra-uterine period of life, at delivery, and during early childhood contributed to deviations such as cerebral palsy, epilepsy, mental defect, behaviour disorders, hyperactivity, reading difficulties and tics. Other workers have attempted to repeat this work and although the final situation has still to be evaluated, there is little evidence that birth factors play a major part in the causation of delinquency, a finding which has been confirmed by the recent longitudinal London study by West and his colleagues, who have also demonstrated that pathologically clumsy children tend to be of limited intelligence and when they displayed delinquency it was the intellectual limitation, rather than the clumsiness, that was the important predictor of the delinquency.

In America shortly before the outbreak of the Second World War, it was planned to carry out a prospective survey of children thought likely to become delinquent. One group was to have counselling and the other was to be used as a control group. This was known as the Cambridge-Somerville Youth Experiment. Due to disruption related to the war, the main aims of this study were not fulfilled, but much valuable information was collected and the McCords followed up youngsters recruited for the experiment. They found that of all physical illnesses and abnormalities, only acne and definite neurological handicap correlated significantly with delinquency. The question of neurological handicap presents many problems in terms of definition and evaluation of the degree of disability. In addition to their neurological handicap, many of these children acquire a secondary social handicap since, because of the nature of their infirmity, they become increasingly dependent on their parents and others in their environment. Because of their disorder, many of these youngsters will have had a prolonged sojourn in hospital with varying degrees of associated deprivation. Rutter and his co-workers examining children with organic brain dysfunction on the Isle of Wight noted that, although they were more susceptible to psychiatric disorder, there was no specificity about the type of disorder, and they were not particularly likely to develop a conduct disorder.

A Swedish follow-up study reported on the outcome of head injuries sustained by one of each pair of a series of twins, which suggested that there was often an exaggeration of previous personality traits and any psychological disturbance was more closely related to this than to the nature of the injuries sustained. The final evaluation of the role of the physical factors, in particular neurological difficulties, has still to be made, but to date there is little evidence to support such factors as being specifically important in the development of conduct disorders and delinquency. In contrast to reports from the earlier parts of this century, it has been shown that, overall, young delinquents are an extremely healthy group.

Whilst a high proportion of adult offenders have a history of mental disorder, there is comparatively little evidence that psychiatric disorder is a contributory factor in the younger age group. Dr. Pamela Mason, surveying admissions to a boy's classifying school, found that only 0·2 per cent had a frank mental illness. But Drs. Cowie and Slater, in a study of girls in a classifying school, and Dr. Peter Scott reporting on a group of approved school boys, all comment on the high proportion of delinquents with abnormal personality traits. Dr. Scott comments on immaturity, sensitivity, apathy, withdrawal and difficulty in making relationships.

In summary, there is little evidence that physical or mental illness by itself is important as an aetiological factor in the development of a delinquent pattern of behaviour in a given individual. However, illness or handicap may be focussed on, and may influence, developing patterns of behaviour in the youngsters so it is important that any recognisable defects should be treated early, insofar as this is possible.

It has been noted that delinquency has been associated with other disorders, particularly enuresis and poor academic attainment. Is it possible that factors inhibiting the learning of bladder control and academic skills also contribute to difficulty in learning socially-acceptable behaviour? Since our knowledge of causative factors in all these areas is minimal, it is not possible to answer this question. It is, however, recognised that many delinquents give a previous history of enuresis, poor reading skills and truancy. It may be that we ought to identify this vulnerable group at an earlier stage and make special educational provision for such children, thus accepting that some young people may have disabilities which make learning more difficult for them than for many other children.

The learning environment
The learning environment may be subdivided into the material environment, the emotional environment and the cultural environment.

It has long been recognised that delinquency occurs more commonly in deteriorated neighbourhoods and in urban rather than rural communities, in association with sub-standard housing, overcrowding and low family income. Yet it is still the individual home which is most important in the final analysis.

The delinquent is more likely to be one of a large family in which the bread-winner is periodically unemployed. Often, there is a broken home and in this context is seems that separation, desertion and divorce are all more significant than loss of a parent by bereavement, it being surmised that prior to the break-up of the parental union there has probably been a prolonged period of disharmony, with arguments, squabbling and verbal and, sometimes, even physical abuse. West, in his recent London survey, comments on the global impression of family conflict in relation to delinquency.

Child-rearing attitudes have also been examined by many workers and over-permissiveness, rigid discipline and inconsistent control have all been implicated at various times as background factors in anti-social conduct. Just as parents have to instruct their children about toilet training, so they must also teach them control of social behaviour. This may be by direct control, initially imposed by the family, later school, and, eventually, by society. By the time the child reaches the age of criminal responsibility at 10 years he should be aware of what forms of behaviour are unacceptable. Ideally, by that age, a child will have developed a system of internalised control and will conform on this account, rather than through fear of discovery of aberrant behaviour. As discussed in the first chapter withdrawal of parental affection is more likely to bring about internalised control and strong conscience-formation rather than erratic discipline and little overall supervision. In general, authoritarian attitudes are not helpful in enabling a child to develop its own, rationally-directed control system.

The cultural environment has also been recognised as playing a causative part in delinquency in certain areas of each community which are known to have a particularly high crime rate. Often this occurs where families in deprived circumstances have tended to congregate.

From what has been said in this section it should be apparent that in the present state of knowledge relatively little can be done about improving the individual's capacity to learn. Preventive work will therefore have to be aimed at improving the learning environment.

Prognostic classification

Very few long-term studies in the field of delinquency have been aimed at identifying prognostic factors associated with this form of behaviour and there is a great need for more prolonged studies to look at the future careers of juvenile delinquents. Gibbens and Silbermann followed up a series of 300 prisoners, comparing them with 100 ex-prisoners applying for after-care. The striking feature was the relationship between personality characteristics and the age of onset of a criminal career. Only a minority of the adult offenders had juvenile convictions and between a quarter and a third had their first convictions after the age of 21. This and other evidence suggests that the positive, aggressive, outgoing person is more likely to be come involved in juvenile crime and that it is the passive, inadequate individual who starts later in life and then continues on a delinquent path as the adult recidivist.

Pritchard and Graham examined the case records of the patients admitted to an adult psychiatric hospital and who had previously been treated in a child psychiatric unit and found that the child who had a behavioural problem tended to become the adult who was treated for personality difficulties. The child with neurotic symptoms became the adult receiving treatment for neurosis, so that there seemed to be some consistent diagnostic 'follow-through' from child to adult life.

Perhaps the most outstanding long-term follow-up study has been that of Robins, who examined 500 child psychiatric patients some 15 years after their episode of illness. She noted that about half the children who had presented with repeated episodes of anti-social behaviour occurring in school, home or the community and with at least one juvenile court appearance, became psychopathic and very few adult psychopaths had not shown some such type of behaviour in childhood.

Treatment classification

It may seem strange, but there were certain illnesses which were cured long before the cause was known, for example, the treatment of scurvy among sailors by the provision of fresh lime juice and the control of cholera by the removal of the handle of the Broad Street pump. These were empirical approaches, carried out long before vitamin C or the cholera organism had been identified. However, the 'cure' for delinquency has proved singularly elusive despite the prolonged search. Recently, we have seen a move away from punitive care to custodial care in an environment with a more therapeutic approach. The so-called 'therapeutic community' is a relative commonplace today, but a definitive solution is still awaited.

One attempt to look at the management of children with conduct disorder was embodied in a report by the London Boroughs' Associations' Working Party on the Provision for Seriously Disturbed Adolescents. This group reported in 1967 and it recognised that three major problems existed. They were:

1. Lack of facilities and lack of co-ordination between those few that were available.
2. Failure to classify adolescents in a way that takes account of the total needs of the disturbed youngster.

3. A tendency to expect too much from psychiatry.

It suggested that in the management of disturbed adolescents some degree of control is needed and that this should be a part of the framework within which treatment is offered. Control can thus be seen as a positive therapeutic measure and permits a classification for treatment according to the degree of control required. In fact, this concept can be elaborated. From it, one can decide whether the child should remain in the community under supervision, or whether removal from home may be necessary. In the latter event, the type of placement should be selected according to the degree of control required. This aspect of management is considered further in Chapter 20.

One of the most ambitious attempts to provide a sub-classification of delinquency is that of Dr. Peter Scott, the well-known forensic psychiatrist. In this he attempts to bring together descriptive, aetiological, prognostic and therapeutic factors and he recognises four groups:

1. The individual well-trained to anti-social standards, taught from childhood to get what he wants without consideration for others. The anti-social behaviour is thus motivated towards material gain. Treatment is seen as consisting of re-training, advising, assisting, befriending and attempting to instil a less anti-social pattern of behaviour through positive relationship. Scott suggested a background of sanctions, if necessary, to help these youngsters.

2. 'Reparative' behaviour where the motivation is emotional gain and the offences are aimed at enabling the individual to adjust to difficulties in his environment: for example, aggressive outbursts may compensate for feelings of inadequacy and inferiority. Recognition of the emotional gain element is necessary to understand this type of offence and treatment involves a basis of sanctions and psychotherapy, so that the delinquent can acquire an understanding of the background to his behavioural pattern.

3. The badly-trained delinquent, where childhood upbringing has been associated with parental inconsistency and poor identification models so that the youngster had inadequately developed internal controls and is himself rather inadequate, tending to become involved in offences which have been suggested by others. The poorly-developed personality makes management difficult and

while sanctions may be useful, if they are too heavy they defeat
their object. Long-term, patient supervision is required in this
group.

4. What Dr. Scott calls the 'Rigid Fixation' group, a mal-adaptive
type of delinquency characterised by repeated, almost self-punitive
offences which are often committed alone.

This is a very sophisticated classification and obviously requires
a diagnostician/therapist who has considerable experience with
young offenders in order to make use of it. However, even for those
coming new to the field, it is valuable in contributing to a better understanding of delinquent behavioural patterns.

Other attempts have been made to classify offenders. In his recent London study, West found that delinquent boys drank more,
smoked more and gambled more than those who did not become
delinquent. From an early age they were noted to be unpopular
with their class-mates and teachers commented on their untidiness,
laziness and defiance.

At a different level, Hewitt and Jenkins identified a group of
socialised (adaptive) delinquents where the individual's personality
appeared to be relatively normal, but where the home circumstances were associated with over-crowding and a degree of
material deprivation, so that the socialised delinquent tended to
spend his time with a local gang. Here, offences tended to occur
outside the home, in contrast to the unsocialised or mal-adaptive
delinquent who showed evidence of impaired personality development, having difficulty with interpersonal relationships and tending
to be unpopular, moody and sullen. This latter type of personality
was found to be associated with rejection by both parents, particularly the mother, whereas the socialised delinquent tended to
have an affectionate mother, although parental discipline often
seemed to be lacking. Unfortunately, attempts to confirm this
classification have not been satisfactory and even in the original
work it was found that a number of children did not fit into either
category.

The Grants developed a fairly sophisticated classification using
the theoretical concepts of Piaget and of Erikson. They felt that
maturity of personality could be identified and they described seven
stages in its integration. At the very lowest level the personality is

so poorly developed that the individual is unable to survive in the outside world. Conversely, those with the highest integration levels are unlikely to be met with amongst a delinquent population and it is the middle levels (stages two to five) which are encountered most commonly with a history of varying degrees of delinquency.

At the beginning of this century we were able to develop a concept of 'mental age' related to the level of intellectual ability and attainment of an individual. Nowadays it seems possible that we may be able to evolve a means of measuring 'emotional age' based on measurements of social learning and achievement.

At the present time, the age of consent is linked to chronological age, but perhaps it may come about that we shall gain responsibility for our behaviour as we attain a defined emotional age. Life is becoming increasingly complex and, as things stand, we are making almost intolerable demands on many individuals, because we thrust responsibility upon them at some arbitrary stage of life. A proportion of what we call 'behaviour disorder' seems to be a reaction to this type of situation and our civilisation needs to consider whether there are not better ways of easing people into an adult pattern of behaviour than the ones we currently employ. It is difficult to avoid appearing paternalistic here, but experience does seem to suggest that emotional maturity and self-control do come to different individuals at different ages. Delayed maturation can cause great difficulties to the individual and to society alike and it seems sensible to consider ways in which the emotional 'slow developer' can be protected from excessive social pressure, so as to prevent possible anti-social backlash.

THE MANAGEMENT OF DELINQUENCY AND CONDUCT DISORDER

Psychiatric involvement with the delinquent or conduct-disordered child is in the first instance at the stage of assessment and diagnosis. The psychiatrist will be particularly concerned to examine the individual's capacity to learn and to discover any disease process which has been interfering with learning. He will also be aware of the importance of the learning environment. Thereafter the further management of the conduct-disordered child may be undertaken by the psychiatrist, social worker, probation officer and/or the educationalist. The Juvenile Court may or may not be involved, and in some instances, it may be the Juvenile Court which institutes assessment procedures, including a psychiatric report.

The Juvenile Courts are special Magistrates Courts at which, except in exceptional circumstances, persons under 17 are tried. The bench consists of lay magistrates and must include a man and a woman with special experience in dealing with children. In the Juvenile Court the punitive role is subordinate and the court has a statutory duty to take into account the needs relating to the welfare of each individual found guilty. The magistrates may request social-enquiry reports from social workers and can ask for a report from a psychiatrist where it is indicated. These reports may be furnished whilst the youngster resides at home, but in some instances an 'interim care order' may be made, usually for a period of three weeks. Under this order the juvenile may have to reside at a local authority assessment centre (formerly a remand home) for observation and preparation of these reports. Although the interim-care order is not intended to have a punitive function, many youngsters interpret it as being 'put away' and regard it as a penal procedure and in some instances this may be quite salutory.

Many of the sanctions available to the magistrates at a Juvenile Court are the same as those in adult Court but in addition there are special sanctions for juveniles. The most commonly used are:

1. *An absolute discharge* (*i.e.,* no strings attached)
2. *A conditional discharge*, which means that no action is taken in relation to the offence of which the youngster was found guilty but should he offend again within a given period, for example, one or two years, this offence may be taken into consideration when he appears subsequently in Court.
3. *A fine.* Usually it is the parent who pays the child's fine, although the magistrate may order that the parent is to be repaid by the juvenile. In an area where work is available at weekends and after school hours, a fine may be of value but where a family is at bread-line level and a child is too young to earn, the debt incurred may be an intolerable burden, so the juvenile may be tempted to steal in order to pay off his debt and very little is achieved. On the other hand, for the young wage earner a fine may bring about the result intended.

4. *Supervision orders.* These were introduced with the 1969 Children and Young Persons Act and replaced the former probation orders. Local authority social workers oversee all youngsters under the age of 14 on supervision orders. Fourteen to seventeen year-olds may be supervised either by social workers or probation officers, but eventually the intention is that all supervision orders imposed by Juvenile Courts will be administered by social workers. Certain conditions may be attached to the supervision order; for example, a youngster may be requested to reside at a given place whilst under such an order and this could be at home, with a particular adult who is willing to have him, or in a hostel. This is known as a 'supervision order with a condition of residence'. Sometimes psychiatric treatment may also be a condition of a supervision order, providing the youngster consents to this, and this may be undertaken either as an out-patient or as an in-patient. The name of the doctor treating the patient or the clinic at which he will be treated has to be declared and a psychiatrist making the recommendation must be recognised under Section 28 of the Mental Health Act 1959. Whilst under a supervision order, the juvenile remains in contact with the supervising professional worker who is able to sort out reality problems and who may help him to progress in his emotional development by means of case work. Co-operation with the social worker is required and he can be brought back before the Juvenile Court for a breach of a supervision order. Should he fail to co-operate, on re-appearance in Court, the original offence would be taken into consideration in addition to the breach of supervision order when considering management.

5. *Attendance centres.* These were introduced under the Criminal Justice Act 1948, being developed from the idea that if juveniles got into mischief in their leisure time perhaps they would benefit from supervised leisure activities. Attendance centres are usually run by the police and some function as small single-sex youth clubs. The maximum time to be spent at an attendance centre is 24 hours and this is usually taken at two-hourly sessions on Saturday afternoon. It is anticipated that attendance centres will be phased-out as intermediate treatment is developed through the implementation of the 1969 Children and Young Persons Act.

6. *Detention centres.* These are also likely to be phased out. They were introduced under the Criminal Justice Act of 1948, with a view to helping the offender from a good home background who

did not respond to a non-custodial sentence. Offenders aged 15 to 21 years can be sent to a detention centre for three to six months. The regime is associated with strict control and the day is fully organised, with emphasis on physical exercise and manual labour so it is only those youngsters who are physically fit who can be considered for a detention centre. Many juveniles have a positive attitude to a period at a detention centre and feel that they have been 'properly punished'. Recently, there has been increased pressure for places at detention centres following the introduction of:

7. *Care orders*. These were introduced under the 1969 Children and Young Persons Act, replacing the former 'Fit Person Order' (by which a juvenile could be committed to the care of a 'Fit person' usually the local authority) and Approved School Order. Now, if the Court sees fit, a juvenile may be committed directly to the care of the local authority. Normally a Care order is in force until the individual's eighteenth birthday but if it is imposed at or after the age of 16, or in other exceptional circumstances, it may remain in force until the person concerned is 19. Once the Care Order is made the local authority has to decide how the youngster under its provisions may best be helped. In some instances, and particularly if there is pressure on places, the youngster may remain at home 'on trial'. Sometimes he may go to a special assessment centre for children under Care Orders, so that the type of residential placement most suited to his needs can be decided upon. A proportion of children under Care Orders go to children's homes, while some go to schools for the maladjusted and others to the former approved schools which are now absorbed into the local authority range of community homes. These residential establishments are described further in Chapter 20.

8. *Borstal training*. Under certain circumstances, juveniles having had their fifteenth birthday may be sentenced to Borstal training. This is happening with increasing frequency at the present time since if an individual, perhaps already on a Care Order and at a Community Home, offends again, there is little that the court can do other than sentence him to a detention centre or recommend Borstal training. With certain particularly refractory delinquents, the court sometimes has little option but to recommend Borstal training. This is particularly ironic, as those who were involved in

framing the 1969 Children and Young Persons Act had envisaged that Borstal training for the under-seventeens could be phased out. Unhappily, with the marked increase in violence and vandalism in recent years, this is not likely to happen in the immediate future. It is important for those professional workers who become involved with delinquent youngsters to have a knowledge of the powers and the functions of the Juvenile Court so that Court involvement can be used in a positive rather than a negative way. But whether or not there has an appearance in Court or Juvenile Court, the youngster needs help to alter his maladaptive pattern of behaviour. Sometimes this will involve case work or psychotherapy and in addition, behaviour therapy methods may be used in some instances. The reader is referred to the relevant chapter for fuller details of these approaches. Group therapy has been used recently with apparent benefit in some residential establishments and also by some supervising, professional workers in a non-residential setting.

REFERENCES AND FURTHER READING

Cowie, J., Cowie, V. and Slater, E. *Delinquency in Girls.* Institute of Criminology, Cambridge, Heinemann, 1968.

Gibbens, T. C. N. and Silberman, M. 'The Inadequate Recidivist.' Proc. R.S.M., 1965, *58*, 705.

Graham, P. and Rutter, M. 'Psychiatric Disorder in the Young Adolescent: A Follow-up Study.' Proc. R.S.M., 1973, *66*, 1226.

Grant, M. Q. *Interpersonal Maturity Level Classification*; *Juvenile.* Community Treatment Department of Youth Authority, March, 1961.

Hewitt, E. E. and Jenkins, R. L. *Fundamental Patterns of Maladjustment.* Springfield, Ill., Michigan Child Guidance Inst., 1946.

*London Boroughs Association. Interim Report of Working Party on *The Provision for Seriously Disturbed Adolescents,* June, 1967.

Mason, P. *The Nature of the Approved School Population and its Implication for Treatment* in *Residential Treatment of Disturbed and Delinquent Boys.* Ed. R. F. Sparks and W. R. G. Hood (Cropwood Conference) Institute of Criminology, Cambridge, 1968.

McCord, W. and McCord, J. *The Origins of Crime.* Columbia University Press, New York, 1959.

Pritchard, M. and Graham, P. 'An Investigation of a group of patients who have attended both the child and adult departments of the same psychiatric hospital.' Brit. J. Psych., 1966, *112*, 603.

Rich, J. 'Types of Stealing.' Lancet, 1956, *1*, 596.
Robins, L. N. *Deviant Children Grown-up.* Williams and Wilkins, 1966.
Rutter, M., Tizard, J. and Whitmore, K. *Educational Health and Behaviour.* Longman, 1970.
Scott, P. D. 'Medical Aspects of Delinquency.' Hospital Medicine, 1966, *1*, 219.
Scott, P. D. 'Delinquency.' Ch. XVI in *Modern Perspectives in Child Psychiatry,* Ed. J. G. Howells. Oliver & Boyd, 1965.
Scott, P. D. *Problems of Deviant Social Behaviour in Delinquency.* Supplement to the British Journal of Psychiat., May 1974, p. 14.
*Scott, P. D. 'The Role of the Psychiatrist in Assessing the Criminal for the Court.' Brit. J. Criminology, 1960, *1*, 116.
Scott, P. D. and Khan, J. H. *An XYY Patient of Above Average Intelligence as a Basis for Review of the Psychopathology, Medical and Legal Implications of the Syndrome and Possibilities for Prevention.* In *Psychopathic Offenders.* Paper Presented to Cropwood Round Table Conference. Ed. D. J. West, Inst. of Criminology, Cambridge 1968.
Sullivan, C., Grant, M. Q. and Grant, J. D. 'The Development of Interpersonal Maturity: Application to delinquency.' Psychiatry, 1957, *20*, 4.
Tutt, N. *Care or Custody.* Darton, Longman & Todd Ltd., 1974.
*West, D. J. *The Young Offender.* Pelican, 1967.
West, D. J. *Present Conduct and Future Delinquency.* Heinemann, 1969.
*West, D. J. and Farrington, D. P. *Who Becomes Delinquent?* Heinemann, 1973.
Williams, D. 'Neural Factors related to Habitual Aggression.' Brain, 1969, *92*, 503.

* *Recommended selected reading.*

11 Personality disorders

As described in Chapter 1, personality development is contributed to by genetic factors and environmental factors. In our present state of knowledge there is little we can do about the more subtle forms of abnormal inheritance, so understandably most work has been concentrated on environmental factors. Many professional workers in the last hundred years have been examining possible theories of personality development, with especial emphasis on stages of intellectual, social or emotional development, according to the particular interest of the professional worker concerned. Perhaps it is unfortunate that theories have developed in isolation and that those interested in emotional aspects of personality development have given little consideration to cognitive functioning and vice versa. In a text of this nature it is not possible to consider any theory of personality development in great depth and so the reader is referred to the appropriate literature, but brief mention will be made of some relevant theories.

THEORIES OF PERSONALITY DEVELOPMENT

Psychoanalytic theory
It is interesting that psychoanalytic theories of personality development arose from the psychoanalysis of adult patients, and yet it is

probably child psychiatrists who have been in the best position to appreciate their relevance. Sigmund Freud is, of course, regarded as the father of psychoanalysis and he saw the mind as having three main components, namely:

1. The id—a mass of instinctual drives and impulses requiring instant gratification. At birth, the infant is regarded as being completely egocentric or id-ridden, demanding immediate satisfaction of primary drives such as hunger. The individual is largely unaware of such drives which are generated within the unconscious.

2. The ego—this is mainly conscious and is associated with the realities of day-to-day living, modifying the demands of the id and being influenced by the superego. Many professionals who may not subscribe to psychoanalytic theory will use terms derived from Freudian theory such as weak ego-strength, impairment of ego-boundaries, etc.

3. The super-ego—this is unconscious, but exercises some control over ego-function and is regarded as equivalent to conscience.

Freud became aware of the pleasure associated with bodily function and at one stage he saw a sexual connotation in this. He recognised that infantile gratification was related to various pleasurable bodily sensations and identified three phases of development in infancy:

1. *The oral phase.* This he regarded as lasting through the first eighteen months of life, the infant's pleasure being associated with gratification of its oral needs, such as feeding, and sucking. If these demands are not met, the infant is likely to become concerned and signals his distress by crying.

2. *The anal phase.* This overlaps and continues from the oral phase until the age of three. During this period, certain social demands (as discussed in Chapter 9) are made on the infant in that he is expected to gain control of bladder and bowels. This is the first time the child is in a position to co-operate actively and it is then that habits like cleanliness, punctuality and tidiness are inculcated with some expectation of success.

3. *The genital phase.* This is associated with the Oedipus complex in boys and the Electra complex in girls, the names being derived

from Greek literature. It is recognised that at this stage the child tends to identify with his parents, particularly the parent of the same sex. Following on from this, the boy may unconsciously feel that he is in love with his mother, so his father is seen as a rival and the boy becomes angry towards his father. He then becomes afraid that his father will be aware of the situation and may punish him by castration. The term 'castration anxiety' has been suggested and Freud proposed that this fear is reinforced by the developing boy's awareness of the female lack of a penis. A counterpart situation in girls has been described as a 'penis-envy'. Freud considered that the genital phase was followed by the *latency period*, a time of relative sexual quiescence, ending about the age of twelve with the onset of puberty.

Puberty and adolescence

While Freudian theory is no longer a predominant influence in the practice of child and adolescent psychiatry, some knowledge of the concepts of psychoanalysis is valuable. At the very least, Freud has stimulated considerable investigative work, even if only by the controversy which he created. To a certain extent, his theories may have been appropriate for the culture in which he was working, though less appropriate to other cultures. An interesting book by Bruno Bettelheim, *The Children of the Dream* describes child-rearing practices in the Israeli Kibbutzim, where sibling rivalry is probably more important than the oedipal situation. From such writings one is made aware of the somewhat culture-bound aspects of some of Freud's work.

Erikson's work

Erikson has built on Freudian theory and has described the maturation stages of man, suggesting that in early infancy the child's relationship with his mother in the feeding situation is crucially important in determining his future attitudes and it is at this stage that trust develops. Should his relationship at this stage be unsatisfactory, he will experience a predominance of mistrust.

It has been proposed that some prominent features in those with personality defects may be generated as a result of emotional fixation at certain stages of personality development. Erikson considers that fixation of personality at an infantile level will result in either a craving for dependency throughout life, the dependency being virtually insatiable, or a rejection of dependency, with resistance to any attempt to gratify dependency needs. The identification with dependency he terms a 'positive' fixation and the rejection of dependency a 'negative' fixation.

As a toddler the child is expected to acquire certain social skills. The control of bowel and bladder function (as outlined in Chapter 9) requires a considerable degree of co-operation from the child, and Erikson views co-operation as the hall-mark of this stage when the toddler develops autonomy. But it is also a period which is associated with temper tantrums in relation to feelings of frustration. Parental control and dominance often become more apparent and this may prove frightening to the developing child. On the other hand, parents may not be sufficiently firm, thus depriving the child of guidelines for its behaviour. Erikson suggests that satisfactory passage through this stage should be associated with developing confidence, whereas shame and doubt arise if it has been an unsatisfactory experience.

In the third stage, which corresponds to Freud's genital stage, the child becomes increasingly aware of his sexual role and his position within the family. In Western culture, he probably makes his first excursions away from home at this time. Erikson sees this as a period when initiative and a lively curiosity develop, but if difficulties arise now the child may become anxious, inhibited and withdrawn, with associated guilt feelings.

Corresponding with the latency period, Erikson describes an age of industry. Here the demands of school and play increases and if this stage proves unsatisfactory, the danger is a lasting sense of inadequacy and inferiority.

In adolescence, Erikson sees the individual's task as the establishment of his own identity. He has to come to terms with who he is, what he is, and where he is going in life. Is he being too ambitious or can he easily achieve his desired goal, or should he even have a goal at which to aim? The emotional problems confronting the adolescent were outlined in Chapter 2 and, as we know, the adolescent has to adjust to the bewildering changes in his body and his emotions, moving from the relative security of childhood to meet the unknown challenge of the adult world. At the same time, many teenagers need to question what were previously acceptable adult standards and values and they may experiment with a variety of behaviour.

For many adolescents, this is a period of emotional turmoil but many professionals working with adolescents feel that equal, or even greater, concern should be manifested towards the over-conforming teenager. The term 'identity crisis' has come to be used to describe this period of turmoil and certain patterns have become recognisable. There is the fortunate adolescent who achieves an identity without any obvious emotional struggle and has a clear goal. Another may have a period of questioning and rebellion, but he and his family may be able to contain the situation so that outside help is not required. Those teenagers who get into major difficulties may experience what Erikson has termed 'role diffusion', lacking a sense of purpose, experimenting with deviant behaviour, or retreating into a fantasy life, and it is for these youngsters that professional help is most often sought.

In young adulthood, the individual's major achievement is associated with the attainment of social intimacy and the major defect is likely to be isolation.

Learning theory

This is based on the premise that behavioural reactions are largely learnt, with modification in behavioural patterns resulting from experience. The use of learning theory in the treatment of abnormal behavioural patterns is discussed further in Chapter 19. Without dignifying their methods with a name, many parents make use of the concepts of learning-theory in an elementary way in their child-rearing practices, in that they often reward socially acceptable behaviour or withdraw approval when socially unacceptable behaviour is manifested. It has been suggested that those children who respond readily to such measures, that is, those who are easily conditioned, tend to develop introvert personalities, whilst those who have difficulty in modifying their behaviour are more likely to become extroverts. This difference in the ease of conditioning may be associated with inherited factors.

Whilst psychoanalytic and learning theories and Piaget's views of cognitive development increase our understanding of some aspects of child maturation, they do not provide a complete answer, and a great deal of research has yet to be carried out before we can talk confidently about personality development.

PERSONALITY DISORDER

To recognise personality deviation, one must be familiar with the normal. Here, the normal may be conceived of as the ideal personality, or alternatively, it may be an individual whose personality is statistically close to the mean. Since personality development continues throughout childhood and adolescence, strictly, one cannot speak of personality 'disorders' until the adult personality has been formed. It is usual, therefore, to avoid making a diagnosis of personality disorder under the age of twenty-five. The aim of child and adolescent psychiatry is to monitor the developing youngster's emotional progress, much as the paediatrician monitors the child's physical growth, with a view to preventing marked personality disorder in adult life, but for the present this is largely a pipe-dream. Follow-up studies, few though they are, do suggest that many teenagers in presenting with conduct disorder are later diagnosed as having personality disorders in adult life. Morris, reviewing the progress of shy and withdrawn children seen at a child guidance clinic, demonstrated that only a minority were likely to develop marked personality problems in adult life with consequent serious social isolation.

Largely independent of the work of child psychiatrists and psychologists, adult psychiatrists have developed classifications of the personality disorders seen in adult life. There is no agreed definition, but the Glossary of mental disorders referred to previously suggests that the term 'Personality disorders' refers to a group of more or less well-defined anomalies or deviations of personality, which are not the result of psychosis or any other illness. The differentiation of these conditions is to some extent arbitrary and reference to a given personality disorder will depend largely on the relative predominance of one of several groups of character traits. Included among the personality disorders is the psychopathic personality and, overall, eight disorders are recognised as follows:

1. Paranoid.
2. Affective (cyclothymic).
3. Schizoid.
4. Explosive.

5. Anankastic (obsessive-
   compulsive).
6. Hysterical.

7. Asthenic.
8. Anti-social.

It should be noted that the above terms can often be used to denote personalities which still fall within normal limits. When we talk about personality disorder, we usually imply that part, or all, of the individual's personality is sufficiently deviant to be regarded as constituting an illness.

The paranoid personality
Those individuals who are over-sensitive and suspicious, reacting excessively to normal life-experience and tending to blame their problems on others, individuals with this type of personality may become unreasonably litigious and they form a well-recognised group of professional plaintiffs in legal circles.

The affective (cyclothymic) personality
This occurs in people whose personalities are excessively dominated by a prevailing mood. In some this may be an irritable, depressed mood, in others it may be a persistent gaiety with a marked zest for life and considerable drive, or yet again it may be a repetitive fluctuation from a depressed to a cheerful mood. The individual who is persistently depressed and pessimistic may also be somewhat hypochondriacal. Certain individuals who are unsure of themselves, and appear to have a persistently high anxiety level, are sometimes also regarded as having an affective type of personality disorder. These people may be uncertain of themselves, frequently seeking reassurance, and many of them have high standards for themselves and become distressed if, under pressure of work, they are unable to keep up these standards.

Schizoid personality
This personality deviation is characterised by social isolation and lack of emotional warmth. The marked shyness tends to make it difficult for the schizoid person to develop close friendships, and so he usually tends to be solitary. Some schizoid individuals appear to have insufficient drive to be dissatisfied with their way of life, but

others may be aware of profound loneliness and seek help on this account.

The explosive personality
Here the personality is characterised by instability of mood, the individual affected being prone to sudden outbursts of irritability or rage, resulting in verbal and sometimes physical aggression and a marked tendency to behave impulsively. Anti-social behaviour may result from an outburst of explosive behaviour, but otherwise these are generally respectable members of the community.

The anankastic (obsessive-compulsive) personality
Individuals with this type of personality tend to be perfectionists with high moral standards and strong conscience-formation, so that any lapse from these standards is distressing to them. They are conscientious people who are beset by self-doubt and insecurity. Their tidiness and punctiliousness may be beneficial in many areas of life, but their inflexibility and over-conformity can also create problems for themselves and others.

The hysterical personality
This tends to be more common in women than in men, although Eliot Slater has drawn attention to the need to distinguish hysterical personality traits from femininity! The typical hysteric craves attention, seeking the limelight but tending to over-dramatise any situation. Superficially, she appears to have a degree of warmth but the shallowness of this is rapidly exposed. Hysterics have difficulty in maintaining friendships with either sex. They frequently marry, but there is commonly a history of marital discord with divorce and perhaps re-marriage. Similarly, they make tremendous emotional demands on their children, who are quite unable to understand the vagaries of their mother's behaviour. They typically manipulate situations in the environment which they are subsequently unable to control and may then seek help in a dramatic way, perhaps by taking an overdose of tablets. Unfortunately, whilst this is a request for help, the very nature of the way in which they seek help may mean that they are spurned. By crying wolf too often, the assistance looked for is forthcoming progressively less often.

The asthenic personality

This has also been termed the 'inadequate personality'. Such personalities show a lack of drive and a reduced zest for life and have marked features of dependency. These characteristics often start at an early age, the child having difficulty in coping with the demands of school and later having problems in transition to the work sphere.

Anti-social or psychopathic personality

Overtly, the psychopath may present as a pleasant, co-operative individual, but behind the facade is an unscrupulous person with a history of anti-social behaviour dating back to childhood and adolescence. Like a child, the psychopath needs immediate gratification of his desires; he does not easily accept frustration; and he pursues a particular goal only to change direction. Whatever his protestations, he cannot be consistent. The psychopath goes on repeating his mistakes and he is unable to learn adequately from experience. The psychopath creates situations with which he cannot cope and if for some reason he cannot opt out as usual, he may over-indulge in alcohol or drugs. Behavioural disturbance is seen in all areas of life, showing in his work record, his history of unstable marriages and frequent Court appearances.

The older the personality-disordered individual, the more likely are his abnormal personality traits to be established with little hope of amelioration. As already mentioned, it is rare to label an individual as having personality disorder until his mid-twenties, since it is hoped that he may still be malleable and responsive to environmental pressures until this age.

In general, treatment of personality disorder in the adolescent is by individual or group psychotherapy, either on an in-patient or out-patient basis, depending on the degree of severity and the possible need to separate the adolescent from his environment.

REFERENCES AND READING

Bettelheim, B. *The Children of the Dream*. Paladin, 1971.
Brown, J. A. C. *Freud and the post-Freudians*. Pelican, 1961.
Erikson, E. *Childhood and Society*. Penguin Books, 1965.
Eysenck, H. J. and Rachman, S. J. 'The Application of Learning Theory

to Child Psychiatry. Part I. Personality.' Ch. 6. in *Modern Perspectives in Child Psychiatry*. Ed. J. Howells, Oliver & Boyd, 1965.

H.M.S.O. *Glossary of Mental Disorders* prepared by Sub-committee of the classification of the mental disorders of the Registrar General's Advisory Committee on Medical Nomenclature and Statistics, 1968.

Hall, C. S. and Lindzey, G. *Theories of Personality*. Wiley, N.Y. 2nd Ed. 1970.

McCulloch, J. W. and Prins, H. A. *Signs of Stress*. Macdonald & Evans, 1975.

Morris, D. P., Soroker, E. and Burruss, C. 'Follow-up studies of shy, withdrawn children.' Am. J. Orthopsychiat., 1954, *24*, 73.

Morris, H. H. Jr., Escoll, P. J. and Wexler, R. 'Aggressive Behaviour Disorders of Childhood—Follow-up study.' Am. J. Psychiat., 1966, *112*, 991.

Robins, L. N. *Deviant Children Grown-up*. Williams & Wilkins, 1966.

Schneider, K., *Psychopathic Personalities*. (Trans.) Hamilton, M. W., Cassell, 1958.

Segal, Hanna. *Introduction to the Work of Melanie Klein*. Hogarth Press, London, 1973.

Shaw, C. R. and Lucas, A. R. *Psychiatric Disorders of Childhood*. Butterworth 2nd Ed. 1970.

Sim, M. *A Guide to Psychiatry*. Churchill-Livingstone. 3rd Edition 1974.

Slater, E. 'Diagnosis of Hysteria.' B.M.J. 1965, *1*, 1395.

Wolff, S. *Children under Stress*. Allen Lane, Penguin 1969.

12 Emotional or neurotic disorders

The emotional or neurotic disorders are those abnormalities of emotion which are not accompanied by loss of reality-sense, such as is seen in psychotic illnesses. Symptoms are similar to most people's reaction to environmental stress, but they are greater in degree and may be more prolonged in duration. The patient and/or his family may experience discomfort on account of his symptoms, but the latter are understandable in the light of his basic personality and of the stress which may be causing them. This is in contrast to the psychoses, where the patient's symptoms cannot be understood of themselves and where the underlying personality is eroded.

The sophisticated lay public tends to divide psychiatric disorders into 'nervous breakdown' and 'madness'. For them, nervous breakdown refers to those emotional disorders which have also been termed neurotic disorders or (psycho) neuroses. Neurosis is derived from the Greek *neuro* meaning nerve and *osis* meaning a state or condition, but for many people this became confusing, as they had difficulty in distinguishing 'nervous' illnesses such as poliomyelitis (infantile paralysis) which are due to a structural disease of the nervous system, and functional disorders like these psychiatric conditions where no specific lesion can be defined.

157

THE SIZE OF THE PROBLEM

Throughout the total age-span, emotional disorders are more common in females than in males and this is certainly true in adolescence. It is also known that the incidence of emotional disorder increases from childhood through adolescence into adult life and it is probable that it is this increase which accounts for the inequality in the sex ratio of referrals to psychiatrists. As mentioned earlier, boys are more commonly seen by the child psychiatrist and females by the adult psychiatrist, but figures for the presence of emotional disorder in adolescents are sparse. In the Isle of Wight study, to which reference has been made previously, when children were screened in their last year of compulsory schooling, a prevalence of emotional disorder of 12·9 per cent was recorded. This figure, moreoever, was obtained from both a selected and an unselected population and this should increase its reliability. However, there is a marked need for further confirmatory investigations.

CLASSIFICATION

The neurotic disorders most commonly seen in adolescence are:

1. Anxiety states.
2. Obsessive–compulsive disorders.
3. Hysteria.

1. Anxiety states

Everyone experiences some anxiety in given situations, for example, the teenager taking his first driving test, taking exams or facing up to some major life situation, such as his or her wedding day. In fact it would be abnormal if one did not have *some* degree of anxiety in such situations. The majority of people cope effectively with their concern and, indeed, there is some evidence to suggest that efficiency may be enhanced by a certain degree of anxiety, although we imply the opposite when we say that someone's anxiety has 'gone over the top', referring to a situation where an individual's level of anxiety has risen to such a degree that this functioning becomes inefficient.

By and large, we tend to speak about anxiety in relation to the unknown or vaguely understood situation and reserve the term 'fear' for more obvious dangers such as skirting a precipice or defusing a bomb. As with pain, anxiety indicates a state of 'dis-ease'. Just as pain indicates that all is not well with one's physical health, so anxiety is an indicator of emotional well-being, or the lack of it. Anxiety may be a symptom of other diseases and, for example, a depressive illness is often associated with anxiety. Perplexity is commonly seen in young schizophrenic patients, particularly where the patient still has sufficient insight to be bewildered by the strange experiences he is undergoing. In such situations, anxiety is secondary, but a primary anxiety state is also recognised. Some workers would classify this under the affective disorders whilst other writers place it under the neuroses (or emotional disorders) as is done here. An anxiety state may be classified into acute and chronic forms and further sub-divided, according to the symptoms which predominate, into:

a. Simple anxiety state.
b. Phobic anxiety state.
c. Somatic anxiety state.

Clinical picture
In a simple anxiety state, the patient's degree of anxiety fluctuates from a mild uneasiness to an acute experience of impending doom. Anxiety is said to be 'free-floating', that is, it is not centred on any particular object, in contrast to the phobic anxiety states shortly to be discussed. The patient may experience a sense of oppressiveness and tend to worry unnecessarily. He feels tense and irritable and, if the anxiety is severe, he will have difficulty in concentrating and registering information, so that he may complain of memory difficulty. This is a subjective feeling and, on testing, impairment of memory function is not detected. Many patients have difficulty in getting off to sleep and their sleep is disturbed by vivid dreams of an unpleasant nature, or even by nightmares. Bit by bit, the anxious patient tends to be increasingly pre-occupied with his own life and will resent it when even the slightest external problem impinges on him.

In addition to these emotional phenomena, the patient can also experience physical symptoms. These appear to be related to a disturbance in the function of the autonomic nervous system, particularly over-activity of the sympathetic part of this system. The patient may appear pale, particularly around the mouth (circumoral pallor) and he may complain of dryness of his mouth and of experiencing a feeling of emptiness or 'butterflies' in his stomach. Many anxious patients have chest pain or discomfort and there may be difficulties in breathing, associated with a feeling of choking. Some patients unconsciously overbreathe so that they wash out excessive amounts of carbon dioxide from their bodies and may feel giddy or even lose consciousness as a result. Appetite may be impaired and nausea, vomiting and bowel dysfunction (especially diarrhoea) may occur, while urinary frequency and menstrual irregularity are also common.

Phobic anxiety states
Phobic anxiety is a common occurrence in the pre-school child, but tends to become less marked as age increases. It has been noted that phobias decline more quickly in boys than in girls, so that whilst the fear of animals occurs in equal frequency in male and female children, such fears are largely confined to females in adult life. As a child approaches school age, fears of dogs, other animals and strange objects decrease, but fears arising from the imagination, such as those of the dark and of imaginary creatures increase, and it is only during adolescence that fears related to social situations associated with a heightened self-consciousness and fear of open spaces really develop. Lapouse and Monk carried out a survey of children in Buffalo (N.Y.) and found that 37 per cent of 9 to 12 year olds had at least seven fears. Rutter, in the Isle of Wight study, showed that fears and phobias were not confined to the group of children in whom they diagnosed an anxiety disorder, although they were most common in this group.

Dr. Issac Marks in his monograph, 'Fears and Phobias' defined phobia as a special form of fear which:

i. is out of proportion to the situation,
ii. cannot be explained or reasoned away,
iii. is beyond voluntary control, and
iv. leads to avoidance of the feared situation.

These may be broken down into single phobias (monophobic

anxieties) or more diffuse phobic anxiety states. Phobias may be further defined according to the nature of the fear. There may be specific animal phobias, such as fear of dogs, spiders or snakes, fear of specific situations such as the dark, height, thunder-storms, open spaces (agoraphobia), enclosed spaces (claustrophobia); or fear of specific social situations (social phobias). These are phobias of external stimuli; there may also be phobias of internal stimuli, for example fear of illness, such as cancer or venereal disease, fear of harming oneself or others, or fear of being contaminated, such as is commonly seen in the obsessive-compulsive neurosis to be described below. These tend to be phobias of the consequences of a situation rather than of the situation itself.

Perhaps the commonest type of phobic anxiety seen in adolescence is social phobia. Timid, shy youngsters may find great difficulty in facing up to the need to increase their social repertoire. Reserved adolescents find it difficult to cope with self-service restaurants, coffee bars, or other public situations; some are prepared to go hungry rather than eat in a public place and will walk rather than get onto a crowded bus. As adolescents increase their life experience, many become less insecure and, in a sense, desensitise themselves, but a number are sufficiently incapacitated to require specialist help. Social phobia seems to be closely related to the teenager's vulnerable self-image and the patient appears to be most anxious in the situations where he feels conspicuous and in situations in which he might make mistakes and be exposed to ridicule or criticism.

This is in contrast to agoraphobia, which usually has its onset in adolescence and where again the adolescent may have difficulty in going into public places or, in severe cases, may be unable to go out at all. (Married women sufferers from this condition have been dubbed 'house-bound housewives'.) In agoraphobia, it is thought that it is a pre-existing anxiety which makes it difficult for the individual to cope with public places. The agoraphobic has difficulty in getting to work, in undertaking simple shopping or becoming involved in leisure pursuits. If she forces herself into a feared situation, she develops symptoms of anxiety like those described above, with a sensation of panic, weakness and unsteadiness. Panic attacks are usually relieved when she withdraws from the feared situation and the presence of a relative or friend can often reduce the intensity of the attack. Social anxiety and tension may be present at other times and many may also experience *depersonalisation* or *de-realisation*—acute and unpleasant feelings of strangeness or unreality. When it is predominantly unreality of the self, the term de-personalisation is used and when it is unreality of the outside world, it is de-realisation. The onset of agoraphobia may be quite sudden, relating to an acute panic attack, but the symptoms may be precipitated by repeated unpleasant experiences. The condition tends to run a fluctuating course and can sometimes be very long-lasting if untreated.

Animal phobias frequently have their onset in childhood, and it seems probable that those persisting into adult life often represent exaggerations of 'normal' phobias which have failed to improve. Some of these occur in isolation, the fear of spiders being particularly common, and may be compatible with an otherwise normal personality development.

Somatic anxiety
In this type of anxiety state, symptoms related to one of the body organs predominate. For some patients, the most acute feature of the illness may be palpitations; for another respiratory difficulties. Persistent overbreathing (hyper-ventilation), as already mentioned, is commonly seen in young people in association with anxiety. The biochemical changes resulting from this may cause a feeling of faintness, the patient complains of pins and needles in her hands and feet and if it is sufficiently severe an attack of tetany (severe muscle cramp) may result. This complication tends to be more common in girls than boys.

Most adolescents show some anxiety about their bodily health and some may be concerned that they have developed a serious physical illness. Detailed questioning usually reveals that this is not the case but, rather, that they have developed an excessive concern about their bodily function. Such hypochondriasis is usually transient, but some unduly anxious young people can be quite crippled by it.

Separation of one kind or another is a common cause of concern in adolescence and *separation anxiety* is commonly seen. Many younger children show relatively little reaction to the death or loss of a parent, providing the remaining parent is in a position to maintain security. However, with the conflicts of adolescence towards independence, vulnerable teenagers may become concerned about the health of a surviving parent, and they may be reluctant to allow this parent out of their sight, even to the extent of following them to the toilet. Where circumstances are less dramatic, the dependant adolescent may still be concerned about the parent's whereabouts; if they have gone out to a regular evening meeting but happen to return late, the teenager's anxieties and fantasies will have had free range. He may well have imagined his parents in a street traffic accident, being taken to hospital or pronounced dead, and he continues his fantasies through the funeral and how he will cope with the situation then and afterwards. This may be very vivid, but of course is usually interrupted by the late return of the parents, who were merely delayed by a traffic jam or puncture. On such an occasion, the over-anxious adolescent may exhibit relief by being verbally abusive to the parents.

Occasionally, epidemics of anxiety occur during adolescence. Two such epidemics occurring in school children have been recorded in which overbreathing resulted in dizziness and fainting. This spread rapidly among the pupils at these girl's schools, and in each case gave rise to fears for a time that some highly infectious virus was present. Such epidemics are usually self-limiting.

Management of anxiety states
1. *A detailed history* is the first essential. Whilst describing how his symptoms developed, the patient may become aware of hitherto unperceived precipitating factors, which can then be examined in some detail. Following this, simple reassurance may be appropriate or planned psycho-therapy (*see* Chapter 19), depending on severity.
2. *Drug treatment.* For those patients who respond, this is the most efficient way of treating anxiety. The drugs most commonly used are the minor tranquillisers and sedatives which include:

a. The benzodiazepines such as chlordiazepoxide and diazepam.
b. Other tranquillisers such as meprobamate.
c. Barbiturates.
d. Where there is some associated depression, anti-depressant drugs.

The use of medication in the treatment of psychiatric disorders is considered in detail in Chapter 18.

3. *Behaviour therapy.* Behaviour therapy is found to be of particular value in the treatment of phobic anxiety and various forms of this treatment are available. These are discussed in Chapter 19.

2. Obsessive-compulsive neurosis

This illness is relatively uncommon in adults and even less frequent in children and adolescents, though it does occur. It is characterised by obsessional thoughts and/or compulsions. *Obsessions* are thoughts which the patient recognises to be abnormal, but which he is unable to put out of his mind although they appear to be silly or ridiculous to him. He incessantly tries to get rid of them, but finds that he cannot do so. It is this quality of resistance, allied with insight, which distinguishes obsessional symptoms from other abnormal experiences such as, for example, delusions. *Compulsions* are actions which the patient feels compelled to carry out, although he recognises them to be ridiculous.

Size of the problem

It is difficult to estimate the incidence and prevalence of obsessional illness in the community at large, as the majority of studies show that the patients have had their symptoms for many years before presenting for treatment. It is thought that less than 3 per cent of psychiatric out-patients have obsessional states and probably under 1 per cent of in-patients. In the Isle of Wight study referred to several times already, when 2,199 10 and 11 year-old children were screened, it was noted that four boys and three girls had obsessional features, but it was not considered that any of these children had a fully-developed obsessional disorder of adult type. At one children's out-patient clinic it has been stated that 1·2 per cent of the children attended with obsessive compulsive neurosis.

Clinical picture

At certain stages of development the pre-school child will have many elaborate rituals; he will touch railings as he passes and will carefully avoid stepping on the cracks in the pavement. Should he inadvertently step on a crack, he has a definite sense of uneasiness and may have to go back to 'undo' the wrong action. It has now been established that this behaviour has no sinister psychological significance, as it is appropriate to this stage of personality development. Many adults have superstitions and would become uncomfortable if they walked under a ladder or used a cracked mirror. Yet if they should do so inadvertently, their anxiety level is quickly reduced when nothing untoward happens and they rarely become preoccupied with the supersitition. One controlled survey of adolescent patients showed that an obsessive-compulsive symptom pattern seemed to occur more commonly in a control group than in a patient group. This was potentially an interesting and possibly a significant finding, but a closer examination of the experimental design showed that the difference in symptom pattern was probably the result of an artifact in assessment rather than a genuine difference. When examining the case histories of five patients presenting at a Los Angeles clinic with obsessive-compulsive neurosis, Judd found that the average age of onset of the illness was seven-and-a-half years, with a range from six years four months to ten years and two months. Although many adult patients do not present for treatment until the illness has been present for many years, one-third give a history of onset of symptoms under the age of fifteen years.

The symptoms seen in an obsessional state are identified as:

a. phobias;
b. obsessional thoughts;
c. ruminations;
d. compulsions.

Phobias are the most common of these symptoms and are said to appear in two-thirds of patients who have an obsessional illness. The background to a phobia is usually a fear of contamination, infection, or venereal disease. Some patients may present with a fear that they have swallowed an object, for example, a coin or a pin and, despite reassurance, cannot accept that they have not done so; consequently they spend a long time futilely checking that the pins or coins known to be in their vicinity are still there. This type of uncertainty is known as *folie de doute*. An elaborate pattern of compulsive behaviour may develop from such an obsession. One teenage girl known to the author, although fully informed on sexual matters, was convinced that if she sat down on the seat of a bus that had been recently occupied by a male passenger she might become pregnant. So, although she might enter a virtually empty bus, she had to wait until she saw a woman vacating a seat at the next stop before she could herself take a seat.

Obsessional thoughts are also common. These are ideas, often irrational, which come to the patient's mind and which he is unable to resist. They are also often obscene, very distressing and at variance with the patient's normal background. They may be associated with compulsive symptoms. Obsessional *ruminations* occur when an idea keeps recurring to a patient, so that he is unable to keep his mind on a productive train of thought.

Compulsive rituals are frequent, occurring in about two-thirds of patients: they are probably the commonest of the true obsessional symptoms, but they are often associated with phobias. Checking and washing are the chief forms of compulsive symptom. A teenager going to bed at night may have to undress in a particular order, put his clothes on a chair in a special way and get into bed in a certain sequence. He may involve his family in this, so that it may be necessary for his parents to bring him up a bedtime drink and carry it to a particular side of the bed, meanwhile standing in a special way. Sometimes parents are quite at a loss to understand what is required of them and if the teenager becomes frustrated, verbally aggressive and emotional, a scene may ensue. There may be similarly complicated rituals in relation to bedmaking, dressing, or washing. Other youngsters, in order to pass through a doorway, may have to touch the door or the upright a certain number of times, and books or other objects may have to be kept in a particular order. Should any family member alter the sequence, or disrupt the checking or washing rituals, they are liable to receive a torrent of verbal abuse.

For the adult patient, an obsessional illness is one of the most distressing of all illnesses and his tolerance is stretched to the absolute limit. For teenagers it is quite inexplicable; they become concerned that they may be going out of their minds and yet feel that if they discuss their symptoms, even with another member of the family, they may be told that they are indeed becoming insane, and, therefore, they often carry their burden in isolation. In fact, it is rare for patients with a clear-cut obsessional illness to 'go out of their minds' and it is the fact that they maintain such clear insight into their difficulties which makes the illness so distressing. Obsessional symptoms may occur in other illnesses and a small proportion of patients with schizophrenia may display them. As already discussed, phobias are seen in anxiety states, but these have a different quality from those of the obsessional. In some individuals with a depressive illness, there may be associated obsessional symptoms which clear up when the depressive illness is treated. Compulsive symptoms have also been described with organic brain disease, particularly in encephalitis lethargica, but the quality of these compulsive symptoms differs from those associated with an obsessional illness; very often they have a rote-like, repetitive air and are complicated by features such as intellectual or memory impairment.

Diagnosis
When making a diagnosis of obsessional disorder, one is implying an illness in which obsessions are the main feature and no other recognisable psychiatric or organic disease is present.

Factors associated with obsessional disorders
There is often a family history of obsessional traits in parents and/or siblings. It has been argued that parents who are particularly neat and tidy and who have high moral standards will insist on their offspring acquiring similar characteristics. However, not all the offspring of tidy parents are equally affected and there is sufficient evidence to suggest that, once again, it may be the particular combination of the seed (that is the patient's genetic endowment) and the soil (his upbringing) which is vital. A higher-than-average number of patients who develop an obsessional illness have marked obsessional traits in their previous personality, tending to be somewhat inflexible, conscientious, orderly, over-scrupulous, insecure and demanding high standards of themselves. Given some of these traits, and a fairly strict upbringing, the scene may be set. It has also been noted that patients with obsessional disorders tend to be of good intelligence and this, taken with their personality traits, means that they are particularly valuable in clerical jobs and are often found employed by banks and in the Civil Service, if their difficulties do not become acute.

Other provoking factors have been noted. For example, pregnancy has been noted to be a precipitating factor in the onset of an obsessional illness in some women. In other patients, promotion, bringing increased pressures, has acted as a trigger. Difficulty in coming to terms with aggressive feeling and with psycho-sexual development may be the background to the appearance of an obsessional illness in adolescence.

The course of the illness

In adults it has been observed that about half of the patients with an obsessional illness have a protracted unremitting course, whereas many others have a phasic course. In a follow-up study of a hundred and eighty-seven adolescents treated as in-patients at Bethlem Royal Hospital during a given period, of the nine obsessionals three had done well, three were somewhat precariously adjusted and three were markedly handicapped by their illness; of these last, one had had a leucotomy. To date, follow-up studies have tended to be done on hospitalised obsessionals or out-patients attending an adult clinic, so that one must be guarded when discussing the prognosis for the adolescent with an obsessional neurosis. This is particularly so since it is generally recognised that the longer the duration of the illness the worse the prognosis. It may well be that there is a group of adolescents presenting with obsessional disorder who can remain well for prolonged periods after recovery, and this is certainly the impression of many workers in the field.

Treatment

The fact that the patient has found someone with whom he can discuss his illness and who has some understanding of the phenomena he is describing may in itself bring a certain amount of relief. Many obsessional patients are worse when they are tense, and a reduction of tension in relation to such an understanding attitude may be beneficial. Unfortunately, it is often not justifiable to be over-optimistic about the prognosis, but one can certainly reassure the patient that he is unlikely to become insane. It has been demonstrated that systematic, explorative psychotherapy is usually inappropriate, but supportive psychotherapy may be of value.
Medication The tricyclic anti-depressants, particularly

clomipramine (Anafranil), have been found to be of some use in patients with obsessional disorders. More recently, the use of large doses of clomipramine intravenously has been used with adult patients. Tranquillisers and anxiolytic drugs have also been used (*see* Chapter 18) and may give a good deal of symptomatic relief.

Behaviour therapy This is used in the management of compulsive symptoms and is described in detail in Chapter 19.

Electro-convulsive therapy is of value if obsessional symptoms are secondary to a depressive illness.

Leucotomy is rarely carried out in adolescence, but if it is, the most likely reason is that the patient has a distressing obsessional illness. This procedure is only employed when the patient is severely incapacitated and other treatments have proved unavailing.

3. Hysteria

The concept of the condition we now know as hysteria goes back to ancient times, and the word 'hysteria' is attributed to Hippocrates. It is derived from the Greek for 'sack' or 'womb' and it was thought that hysteria could only occur in women and was related to the wandering of the uterus (womb) through the body, as a result of its becoming desiccated in sexually-deprived women. This theory of hysteria persisted virtually unchanged until the seventeenth century, when the relationship between the brain and hysteria was first contemplated. Today, the concept of hysteria is again under review. The fact that certain individuals under stress react with symptoms of conversion or dissociation is not in dispute, but it is felt that these do not add up to a specific illness but rather occur in relation to other syndromes. Dissociation and conversion symptoms are thought to originate from mental conflict in the absence of organic illness. Conversion symptoms arise when the stress is converted into a physical or mental symptom. It has been suggested that if the conversion of the anxiety arising from the conflict is very complete, the anxiety apparently disappears and the patient presents with excessive blandness, known as *la belle indifférence*. In dissociation, there is an alteration of consciousness in one circumscribed area of experience so that, for example, some patients may wander around in a state of altered consciousness known as a *fugue*. This may be associated with an alteration in memory function and temporary amnesia can occur (*see* below). Until recently, where conversion or dissociation symptoms were present and appeared to be associated with emotional gain, a diagnosis of hysterical illness would have been made. However, the word hysterical has been used so loosely by the lay public, casualty physicians and others, that 'hysteria' has come to be regarded simply as attention-seeking behaviour and has therefore lost its specificity. Practising psychiatrists have become aware that, in recent decades, they are making the diagnosis of hysteria with decreasing frequency, and at times this is mostly an indication that the patient cannot be placed in another diagnostic category and has some 'nuisance value'. It is recognised that hysterical symptoms are more likely to arise at the extremes of life, but also occur to excess in those who are emotionally immature, or who, on account of mental retardation, have a limited capacity to deal with the day-to-day stresses they encounter. It is interesting that, in the Isle of Wight study, Rutter and his colleagues found no cases of hysteria among the young people they studied.

The clinical picture
Obviously this varies with the predominance of particular symptoms. Dissociative symptoms arise as a result of the splitting of consciousness, so that the patient is unaware of inconsistencies in her approach to reality. Common dissociative symptoms involve disorder of memory and disorder of consciousness. Occasionally, an adolescent will hear distressing news such as about the unexpected death of a parent, and may react by developing a severe hysterical amnesia. Usually this memory loss recovers spontaneously after one or two days, even without treatment.

The commonest disturbance of consciousness is the hysterical fugue in which the patient may leave home and wander about for a time in a state of altered consciousness. In this state the patient provides for his basic needs by eating, toileting and sleeping appropriately, while avoiding common dangers. The end of the fugue-like state may be abrupt and the patient is often left with impaired recollection of the period of the fugue.

Conversion symptoms can involve special senses, so that occasionally hysterical blindness or hysterical deafness are seen. Hysterical symptoms involving paralysis or spasms of muscles may also arise, and hysterical convulsive states occasionally present in adolescence. Differentiation of the latter from true epileptic attacks is usually fairly simple, but in some instances proves quite difficult. Fortunately, these highly dramatic manifestations seem to have become relatively rare nowadays.

Treatment
The keystone of treatment is the identification of the stress giving rise to the symptoms and the identification and treatment of any underlying illness. Occasionally, the forms of therapy involving suggestion (such as hypnosis or narcosis) may be required.

Normality and abnormality in childhood and adolescence
In later adolescence the syndromes just described may be fairly well-defined, but in childhood and early adolescence they tend to be much less clear-cut. In a study of adults presenting with neurotic symptoms who had been treated years before at the children's psychiatric department of the same hospital, it was found that having had these childhood illnesses appeared to predispose to adult neurotic symptoms. On the other hand, it has to be said that several studies suggest that children presenting with neurotic symptoms relatively rarely develop severe emotional illnesses in adult life. These contradictory results may reflect differing compositions of the groups under survey.

Some decades ago, it was customary to enquire about so-called neurotic traits in childhood such as thumb-sucking, nailbiting, stammering and enuresis. With a better understanding of child development, it is now recognised that stammering and nocturnal enuresis can be part of the normal developmental pattern. Thumb-sucking is common in young children, and while its persistence may indicate emotional immaturity, there is no evidence that it is associated with a tendency towards adult neurosis. At certain stages in childhood, it would seem that some of the so-called 'neurotic traits' have to be accepted as part of normal development. However, this message takes a long time to get across to the general public and many parents still worry unduly about childish habits which prove to be transient.

In an epidemiological survey of emotional symptoms in childhood, it was noted that the level of parental anxiety was important in the selection of those children who present to the psychiatrist for professional help. Some recent evidence suggests that the daughter of the neurotic mother is more liable to present with neurotic symptoms than is her brother. To what extent this influence is genetic has yet to be elucidated more precisely, but it seems likely that home influence, and perhaps, particularly, patterning of the daughter's behaviour after the mother's example, must have a significant effect.

REFERENCES AND FURTHER READING

Anxiety state

Lader, M. *Studies of Anxiety*. British Journal of Psychiatry. Special Publication No. 3. Headley Brothers Limited, 1969.
Lader, M. and Marks, I. *Clinical Anxiety*. Heinemann, 1971.
Marks, I. *Fears and Phobias*. Heinemann, 1969.
Rutter, M., Tizard, J. and Whitmore, K. *Education, Health and Behaviour*. Longman, 1970.
Woolfson, G. *Recent Advances in Anxiety States* in *Recent Developments in Affective Disorders*. Ed. Coppen and Walk, British Journal of Psychiatry, Special Publication No. 2, Headley Brothers Limited, 1968.

Obsessional compulsive disorders

Berman, L. 'Obsessive Compulsive Neurosis in Children.' J. Nerve and Ment. Dis., 1942, *92*, 26.
Ingram I. M. 'Obsessional Illness in Mental Hospital Patients.' J. Ment. Science 1961, *107*, 382.
Judd, L. L. 'Obsessive Compulsive Neurosis in Children.' Arch. Gen. Psychiat., 1965, *12*, 136.
Mayer-Gross, Slater, and Roth. *Clinical Psychiatry*. 3rd Edition. Ballière, Tindall & Cassell, 1969. Page 126 seq.
*Pollitt, J. 'Obsessional States.' Brit. J. Hosp. Med., 1969, 1146.

Hysteria

Gold, S. 'Diagnosis & Management of Hysterical Contracture in Children.' B.M.J., 1965, 121.
Marks, I. 'Research in Neurosis: A Selective Review 1. Causes and Courses.' Psychological Medicine, 1973, *3*, 46.
Proctor, J. G. 'Hysteria in Childhood.' Am. J. Orthopsychiat., 1958, *28*, 394.
Reed, J. L. 'Hysteria.' Brit. J. Hosp. Med., 1971, *5*, 237.
Rutter, M. L. 'Relationship between child and adult psychiatric disorder.' Act. Psych. Scan., 1972, *48*, 3.
Slater, E. 'Diagnosis of Hysteria.' B.M.J., 1965, *1*, 1395.

* *Recommended selected reading*

Hyperventilation

Enger, N. B. and Walk, P. A. 'Hyperventilation Syndrome in Childhood.' J. Paed., 1967, *70*, 521.

Moss, P. D. and McEvedy, C. P. 'An epidemic of overbreathing among school girls.' B.M.J., 1966, *2*, 1295.

McEvedy, C. P., Griffith, A. and Hall, T. 'Two School Epidemics.' B.M.J., 1966, *2*, 1300.

Normality and abnormality in childhood

Lapouse, R. and Monk, M. A. 'An Epidemological Study of Behaviour Characteristics in Children.' Amer. J. Publ. Hlth., 1958, *48*, 1134.

Lapouse, R. and Monk, M. A. 'Fears and Worries in a Representative Sample of Children.' Amer. J. Orthopsychiat., 1959, *29*, 803.

13 Persistent non-attendance at school

It is only within the last hundred or so years that free full-time education has been available for all children. Under the 1944 Education Act in England, it became the duty of the parent of every child of compulsory school age to cause him to receive full-time education suitable to his age, ability and aptitude, either by regular attendance at school or otherwise. In England, at present, compulsory school age is five to sixteen years.

Absence from school may be for one of the following reasons, or a combination of them:

1. Illness.
2. Parental withdrawal or withholding.
3. Truancy—the pupil is absent without parental consent.
4. School refusal.

The psychiatrist is most frequently involved when truancy or school refusal is suspected as being the cause of a child's non-attendance at school. Tyerman argues that there is little value in distinguishing between truancy and what he calls school-phobia (which is perhaps more logically called school-refusal) but there is some evidence to suggest that until more detailed follow-up studies are available there may be merit in continuing to make this distinction.

SIZE OF THE PROBLEM

It is difficult to obtain accurate figures. The Education Welfare Officers' National Association has carried out surveys from time to time but admits that the problem of definition is great. Many children may be out of school at a given time because of minor ailments, for which the family doctor may or may not be consulted. Recurring absences on account of physical illness may eventually create emotional problems for the child, who finds that he cannot keep up with the work and particularly when his former friends have become involved with other children.

At one time prosecution for non-attendance at school under the 1944 Education Act could give a legal guide to the size of the problem. In some areas it was the practice to take the parent to court in the first instance, when a fine might be imposed. If this did not effect the desired result the erring pupil might then be brought before the Juvenile Court when the outcome could be a supervision order.

With recent legislation, non-school attenders are only brought to Court after consultation with the local authority Social Services Department so that to some extent prosecutions are influenced by the attitudes of this Department. Consequently nowadays Court statistics are even more selective than formerly. Paul Medlicott, writing in *New Society*, has drawn attention to the difficulty in estimating the size of the problem and looks at the current problem in Manchester where 11 to 12 per cent of the school population may be absent on any one day (including those absent for medical reasons). In the same city before the introduction of the Children and Young Persons Act 1969, 350 children were taken to juvenile court each year, but at the time of writing the figure is under 50.

TRUANCY

Truancy is usually defined as unlawful absence from school without the parent's knowledge or permission. The classic truant leaves home at the usual time each morning *as if* to go to school, returning at the end of the school day. A clever truant recalls what he has had for school dinner and knows what homework has to be done for the following day, although he has in reality spent the day out of school on his own, or with others. A few truants at a loose end may get involved with petty crimes, in keeping with the old adage that 'Satan finds some mischief still, for idle hands to do'. Parents usually become aware of a child's truancy as a result of a visit from the Education Welfare Officer, or it may come to light during police enquiries into a delinquent episode. Truancy is more common among boys than girls and occurs most frequently during the period of secondary schooling. It is viewed with considerable seriousness by those in authority, as many delinquents give a history of persistently playing truant as the first hint of a later pattern of anti-social behaviour.

From personal experience, one is aware that one child may be taken before the court after a brief period of absence from school, whilst another may be out of school for a year before action is taken. The kind of action taken may depend on the degree of sophistication of parent, teacher or Educational Welfare Officer. The psychiatrist may become involved at the instigation of the family doctor, or at the request of the Court for a psychiatric report. Incidentally, it is a sad reflection on our time that, where a child is remanded on an interim care order, or the case is adjourned for psychiatric, psychological and social work reports by the Juvenile Court, specialist opinion will usually be forthcoming within three weeks, whereas the same child may languish on the waiting list of a hospital psychiatric out-patient clinic, or child guidance clinic, for a much longer period if the Court is not involved.

The majority of truants are from underprivileged homes. There is often a family history of truancy and, at the least, there is no parental encouragement to achieve academically. The families tend to be large and discipline inconsistent. Father is often absent, or, if present, may be ineffectual.

Recently, Tennent compared a group of boys remanded because of offences under the Education Act with a group of offenders against property, and demonstrated that boys in both groups came from the lower strata of society and from large families with a history of delinquency among the siblings. Both groups had a high incidence of emotional disorder. The only finding of note was that those charged under the Education Act were significantly more often the youngest members of their families. As with many delinquents, truants as a group have poor academic attainments, their reading age being poor despite reasonable intelligence in some cases.

Why do children truant? Earlier studies suggested that truancy was part of a rebellion against adverse circumstances, associated with dissatisfaction with the situation at home and at school. Sociological data available amply confirm that these children have every reason to be dissatisfied with their environment of deprivation. Dr. Harriet Wilson, in her contribution entitled *The Socialization of Children* (in Robert Holman's *Socially Deprived Families in Britain*), details the effect of such an environment so graphically that one wonders if, in this generation, we have over-emphasised the damaging effect of emotional deprivation to the neglect of material and cultural deprivation of the under-privileged. Dr. Wilson has also drawn attention to the fact that children from middle-class homes are educated by teachers who are often from a similar background, so that parent and child can identify with the teacher and the aims of the school, whereas the child from a socially deprived background is in an unfamiliar environment. As time goes on, and as the latter fails to keep up with his age peers in learning to read etc., he becomes understandably discouraged and his motivation to attend school decreases.

Whilst no one would like to put the clock back to the situation where children only moved up to the next class if their attainments were fully acceptable for that class, it does seem as if these children need extra help with basic learning. Designation of priority areas in education should be a help, providing one can find staff of suitable calibre willing to work in these areas, and perhaps an improved teacher/pupil ratio will help to reduce some of the very real frustrations which these children experience. Many of them are self-conscious about their lack of reading and arithmetical skills, but sometimes disguise this with a show of anti-authoritarian aggressiveness.

The availability of basic reading texts with masculine themes appropriate to young teenagers, in place of 'Janet-and-John' type books, should also be a further stimulus for these children. Adolescents who have problems with writing and spelling are only too well aware that this is a form-filling era and that they will almost certainly be asked to complete documents when they start applying for jobs. It is also important for them to be able to read the questions to which an answer on the form is required. One is aware that at this point one is encroaching on the educationalist's field but it is there that this problem can be most profitably tackled.

Under the 1969 Children and Young Persons Act, the persistent truant may be brought before the Court and may be placed on a Supervision Order. If he fails to return to school under supervision and is again before the Court, there is a likelihood that a Care Order will be made. When the Care Order is made, the child is placed in the care of the local authority, but it is normal practice for the Care Order to be supervised by the Social Services Department and not the Education Department. One wonders if an appropriate educational placement might be forthcoming more rapidly, in more cases, if the Education Department had at least some responsibility for the supervision of Care Orders of those who have been 'charged' under the Education Act.

SCHOOL-REFUSAL

School-refusal is defined as persistent non-attendance at school, despite parental encouragement. The child often expresses a desire to return to school and may even get up on a particular morning, dress in school uniform, go out to the bus stop or school entrance, only to realise that he *cannot* go into school. (This is a contrast to the attitude of the truant who will sometimes admit that he *will not* return to school). When first described, this syndrome was referred to as school-phobia but it seems preferable to use the term 'school-refusal', as school-phobia implies an aetiological factor and thus the issue may be prejudged.

Clinical picture
Many of these pupils absent themselves from school for the first time after transfer to secondary education, but others will have had a history of difficulty in settling at infant or junior school and may have been treated for school refusal at an earlier stage of their educational career. If pressurised to go to school, the child has a sensation of fear and may exhibit pallor, especially round the mouth. This fear may be associated with somatic (bodily) symptoms such as butterflies in the tummy, actual abdominal pain or even vomiting, headache or limb pains. Sometimes other

behavioural aspects are also apparent and for example, the child may lock himself in the bathroom or run out of the house. In general, there is an absence of the anti-social symptoms associated with truancy. The onset may be acute or insidious and, for instance, may occur after a child has had a lawful period of absence from school on account of a genuine physical illness, thereafter finding it impossible to return to school when physical health has been restored. Difficulty in getting to school is also most commonly seen after an absence for other reasons, such as the beginning of the new term or following a half-term holiday and, once attendance has been re-established, these should be recognised as vulnerable periods for the future. Symptoms tend to be minimal over weekends and school holidays, only to recur with full severity on Monday mornings, or each succeeding morning that the child is exhorted to return to school. Once it is conceded that the child need not go to school on a particular day, the symptoms recede. Other group activities may be given up at the time that attendance at school ceases. The child may cling to his mother, even following her to the toilet, and may try to prevent her leaving the house or pursue her during her other activities. Unlike truancy where boys predominate, school refusal affects boys and girls in equal numbers and they tend to be of average intelligence, with academic attainments commensurate with their ability. They have often been previously conforming, and have grown up in homes where education is valued—again in contrast to the truant.

Factors contributing to the syndrome
The background to a child's school refusal may occasionally be in the school situation, although more often difficulties at school are merely precipitating factors, drawing attention to more serious underlying problems. Factors are usually multiple but for clarity they will be analysed as if they arose independently.

1. Factors in the school situation may be:
a. *Academic*—where a child's particular problem such as poor reading skills may not be adequately recognised. The teacher may have an awareness of the difficulty, but if this is somehow not communicated to the child, he is apprehensive in case he is asked to

read aloud to the entire class. Occasionally, a highly-intelligent child may become frustrated and 'opt out' of such a situation.

b. *Teacher-pupil relationships.* A sensitive child may feel he is being picked on by a particular staff member. If the situation is recognised and can be talked through, this may be a valuable learning experience for the child.

c. *Peer group relationships.* Why are some children picked on, teased or bullied? Other pupils quickly recognise the youngsters who are not able to stand up for themselves and they take advantage of their weakness. Sometimes the pupil prone to be teased has good friends of his own, who will spring to his defence and the situation is contained, but what happens when the chief defender moves house or school and is no longer available? This sort of problem in relationships with other pupils is a common factor in precipitating absence from school and is usually evidence of other serious underlying relationship problems. This is also the area which is most difficult to help within the school setting, as increased staff surveillance is recognised by the school refuser's contemporaries and this further alienates the child from his own age group.

d. *Pubertal problems.* These may present in the school situation under many guises, but seem particularly common in the insecure girl who has an early menarche and finds such situations as communal showers a problem. On the other hand, a boy with delayed puberty finds himself at a disadvantage in a similar situation.

In all these areas, there may be reality factors, but often the child has an irrational fear and is quite unable to accept reassurance.

2. Factors outside the school

Although aversion to school is normally blamed on problems in the school situation, absence is more often related to problems in the individual and in the home. Some workers feel that the main problem is *separation anxiety*, fear of being away from mother and home being displaced on to school. Many studies comment on the mother-child relationship, the child being over-dependent on the mother and sometimes having been over-indulged. In many instances, there is evidence that this dependence is of long-standing and may, in fact, have been fostered by the mother on account of her own emotional needs. This is particularly likely to arise in a situation where a child has been conceived following a family tragedy; where he is born when other siblings are approaching adolescence, or when he is the only child conceived after years of infertility. Some children, however, show less evidence of long-standing dependence and it would appear that this latter group are unable to cope with normal adolescent pressures towards independence (see Chapter 2). To the vulnerable child, the change from primary school, where each class has a relatively permanent classroom base with one teacher for most of the day, to secondary education (be it secondary modern, grammar or comprehensive school), where classroom and teacher change with each subject, necessitating the movement of large numbers of pupils into the corridors at the same time, is particularly threatening.

Studies of families of school-refusers suggest that mothers have often had neurotic difficulties of their own and this was confirmed by Berg in a recent study. He administered the Eysenck Personality Inventory to the mothers of school-refusers and found that they scored at significantly neurotic levels. In contrast, the school-refusers themselves, with the exception of a group of girls defined as chronic school-refusers, did not score high on neuroticism. In clinical studies, the fathers of school-refusers, although providing well materially for their families, tend to 'opt out' in the home situation, presenting a rather passive, inadequate identification model for the teenager.

Diagnosis
School-refusal, by definition, demands the element of insistence on school attendance by parents and society, so it can never be an independent diagnostic entity. Occasionally, it may be the presenting feature in a psychotic illness, dominated by affective features of anxiety and/or depression. Obsessional symptoms may result in difficulty in functioning at school and because of a child's reluctance to disclose his ruminations or rituals even to his parents, the presenting symptom may be one of school refusal (see Chapter 12). Once specific diagnostic groupings are excluded however, there is still a group of children who cannot go to school and who do not fit into the ordinary classification. These children appear to have difficulty in accepting the demands which school makes on them and have a low tolerance of frustration. Instead of rebelling actively, as the truant does, they react passively and opt out of the

stressful situation. They may be following parental example and in some instances may even be encouraged subtly by a parent. They lack self-reliance and have a poor self-image, so that it appears that temperamental traits play a predominant role in their particular behavioural deviance. One suspects that it is from this group that future work-refusers are largely found.

Management
Initially, this is likely to be in an out-patient setting. All recognisable contributory factors will be explored and if these appear to have a reality basis, where possible they will be remedied. Contact with the school will be established and the child may then be encouraged to return to school. In more serious cases this may need to be associated with a process of desensitisation (*see* Chapter 19), the youngster being encouraged to walk past the school outside school hours, then to enter the school and wander round under supervision, or later to tour the empty school building. Usually a sympathetic escort, a young friend, parent, nurse or other therapist (psychologist or social worker) will have to be involved in these exercises, in order to prevent an upsurge of anxiety in the threatening situation. Some form of medication such as diazepam (Valium) 2 mg, or one of the other anxiolytic drugs described in Chapter 18, may be taken a short while before setting off in order to alleviate anxiety. Once the patient feels at ease in the empty school building, the next stage is to introduce him to the class situation. This may be with an escort as above, or another pupil may take over the role if he feels that an adult companion would make him too conspicuous. Starting with brief periods of 5 to 10 minutes, the length of time spent in the classroom is gradually increased until he is coping with a full timetable.

Many variations of the above are possible. One of the disadvantages in the method just outlined is that the pupil may be introduced to several subjects over a short time and if he has been absent from school for a long time he will be behind on the actual work schedule. So, if a pupil lives near to the school it may be preferable to ascertain his favourite subject and invite him to go to all lessons on that subject during the week, adding one or two additional subjects each week until he is involved in the full curriculum.

Obviously, use of any such method is dependent on the sympathy of the school, but it is rare to have a school fail to give full co-operation if the plan is outlined in advance.

Whilst, efforts to reduce the patient's anxiety are proceeding, the parents must be helped to see their role in the situation and encouraged to support the teenager in his attempt to resume life in the community. They and the teenager should be warned of the risk of relapse, following absence resulting from genuine physical illness or from school holidays.

Where measures such as these are unsuccessful in re-establishing school attendance, boarding-school placement may be appropriate (*see* Chapter 20). Sometimes it is felt that boarding is not suitable and for a minority of school refusers in-patient treatment in a hospital adolescent unit will be required. Many of these units have a school associated with them. However if not, the loss of education can always be made up at a later stage and it is the lack of opportunity to form meaningful relationships with their own age group and the fact that the housebound patient often misses out on social learning which are the main causes of concern. After a period in hospital, when adolescents will be helped in areas of development (*i.e.*, peer group relationships, becoming more independent overall and social learning), the re-introduction to school and the community has to be tackled. At the author's adolescent unit, the majority of school-refusers return to the school of their choice directly from hospital. Local authorities have been extremely helpful in providing bus passes and transport. The regime in use at the time of writing is as follows:

First week—He goes to school from hospital (if necessary escorted by a member of hospital staff) Monday to Friday. If successful, he returns home on Friday directly from school for the weekend. He goes back to hospital on Sunday.
Second week—He goes to school from hospital on Monday to Thursday. If successful he returns home directly from school on Thursday. On Friday, he goes to school from home and returns home for weekend. He goes back to hospital on Sunday.
Third week—To school from hospital on Monday to Wednesday. If successful he returns home from school on Wednesday. On Thursday he goes to school from home again on Friday when he

returns home for the weekend. Back to hospital on Sunday.
Fourth week—To school from hospital on Monday and Tuesday.
If successful, he returns home from school on Tuesday. On
Wednesday, Thursday and Friday he goes to school from home
and returns home on Friday for the weekend.
Fifth week—To school from hospital on Monday and if successful,
he returns home on Monday. He goes to school on Tuesday,
Wednesday, Thursday and Friday from home and stays at home
for the weekend. Returns to hospital on Sunday.
Sixth week—He goes to school from hospital on Monday and is
discharged if all is well.

Inevitably, half-term holidays, inter-current illness or other
events occur to interrupt the above schedule, but despite this, to
date the regime has worked well. Variations are made according to
the needs of the individual child.

Course of the condition
This depends on the factors contributing to the child's difficulties in
coping with school. About one-third, whose problem in school
attendance appears to be associated with features of an inadequate
personality, will almost certainly have similar problems in their
work situation in adult life, or become house-bound housewives. It
is in an attempt to prevent such later repercussions that home-
teaching should be avoided unless the next stage in management is
clear, for example, awaiting a boarding-school place, or awaiting
admission to a hospital adolescent unit as an in-patient or day
patient. It cannot be emphasised too strongly that the majority of
these youngsters have problems in the social rather than the
academic situation.

On the positive side, Dr. Mary Capes, in a five year follow-up
study which examined seventeen school-phobias (as she termed
them), found that work refusal was not a significant later problem
and that a proportion were undertaking further education training.

REFERENCES AND FURTHER READING

Berg, I., Nichols, K., Pritchard, C. 'School Phobia. Its classification and
relationship to dependancy.' J. Child. Psychology and Psychiatry,
1969, *10*, 123.

Capes, M., Gould, E., Townsend, M. *Stress in Youth*. O.U.P. 1971. (Occasional Hundreds No. 1).

Educational Welfare Officers National Association 1965. *For Every Child a Chance*. Unpublished Memorandum.

H.M.S.O. Education Act 1944.

Hersov, L. A. 'Persistent Non-Attendance at School.' J. Child. Psychology and Psychiatry, 1960, *1*, 136.

Hersov, L. A. 'School Refusal.' Brit. Med. J., 1972, *3*, 102.

*Hersov, L. A. 'Neurotic Disorders with special reference to School Refusal' in *Residential Psychiatric Treatment of children*. Ed. P. Baker. Crosby, Lockwood and Staples, 1974.

Medlicott, P. *The Truancy 'Problem'*. New Society 1973. *25*, 768.

Tennent, T. C. 'Truancy and Stealing.' Brit. J. Psychiatry, 1970, *116*, 587.

*Tyerman, M. *Truancy*. University London Press, 1968.

*Wilson, H. 'The Socialisation of Children.' Chapter 3 in *Socially Deprived Families in Britain*. R. Holman. Bedford Square Press, 1970.

* *Recommended selected reading*

14 Anorexia nervosa

This syndrome was described by Gull in this country in 1868 and, independently, in France by Lasègue in 1874. Anorexia nervosa is characterised by:

1. A disturbance of food intake, usually a failure to eat sufficient food, hence the term anorexia, but episodes of over-eating (bulimia) may also occur.
2. Marked weight loss.
3. Disturbance of body image.
4. When appropriate, absence of normal menstrual function (*i.e.*, in females of reproductive years).
5. The absence of a specific disease entity underlying the disorder.

CLINICAL PICTURE

Typically, the history is that of a young girl in her teens or early twenties who has decided to diet, as she is concerned about being overweight. In some instances this is a reality problem, but occasionally the patient may never have been overweight. Dieting continues after satisfactory weight loss has been achieved, and may go on even to the point of emaciation. Many patients state that they feel hungry but cannot eat, and they may feel guilty if they do take food. All fattening foods are omitted from the diet and many patients work out the exact calorie equivalent of their food intake. Sometimes they show excessive zeal in ensuring that members of their family, especially the mother, have a nourishing diet, often with abundance of calories. Patients with this syndrome rarely admit to being ill and, in addition to reducing calorie intake, they may resort to extremes of exercise in order to expend energy and lose weight. The weight loss is secondary to the reduced intake of calories. Whilst it is recognised that starvation may produce disturbance in the menstrual cycle, including amenorrhoea, it is thought that the 'secondary' amenorrhoea associated with anorexia nervosa in girls is of essentially endocrine origin, as in over one-third of patients it coincides with, or may precede, the weight loss. Constipation may be an associated symptom and many anorexic patients resort to purgatives in an attempt to increase weight loss further when, in fact, the symptom is due to sheer lack of food intake. Patients who are normally the most open of people before the onset of the illness, will often conceal food and many induce vomiting in order to accelerate weight loss. Patients have a disturbance of their body image and although still emaciated, become convinced that they are fat. Prolonged mirror gazing in the nude is a symptom which is thought to be of serious prognostic import. This symptom is unlikely to be volunteered and the question will have to be asked directly in order to elicit it. A proportion of anorexic patients steal and there may be a compulsive element in thefts, which appear to be more common during a phase of over-eating; it is often, but not always, food which is stolen.

The physical signs associated with this condition are regarded as secondary to the emaciation and include slowed heart rate, hypotension and a growth of fine downy hair on the trunk and limbs known as lanugo. Hands and feet may be cold and blue (acrocyanosis).

Some workers feel that anorexia nervosa is not a specific entity, but rather that it is the result of an underlying illness such as schizophrenia, serious depressive illness or neurotic illness. Others feel that there may be an anorexia nervosa-like syndrome which is related to another underlying psychiatric illness, but that in addition there is a primary syndrome of anorexia nervosa proper. It is obviously important to establish that there is not an underlying primary psychiatric disorder, and if such is present, treatment is directed towards it in the first instance.

A case of anorexia nervosa has not been recorded from a home where food intake is restricted by economic circumstances. The typical anorexic patient comes from a professional or middle-class background and is of average or above-average intelligence.

FACTORS CONTRIBUTING TO THE SYNDROME

A family history of mental illness has been described in about one-third of patients. Precipitating factors have been examined by many authors. At an early stage, it was considered that sexual conflicts might initiate a preoccupation with weight and body image. Academic pressure has also been considered to be a contributory factor and, in other instances, the illness has followed a teenager's prolonged sojourn away from the bosom of her family, thus bringing her prematurely face-to-face with adolescent drives towards independence. Conflict within the family has also been considered an aetiological factor and some studies have described a parental situation where the mother is the dominating figure with a rather passive father, the affected teenager having a dependent relationship with the mother. Other studies have seen mothers as being rejecting or even normal in their relationships with their offspring. In fact, there is as yet little agreement as to the fundamental causative factors.

TREATMENT

The physical aspects of this syndrome are usually tackled first. Admission to hospital is required for the majority of patients. The aim is to reduce calorie expenditure and to increase the intake of calories. The former is achieved by complete bed rest, which also has the advantage of enabling staff to control the situation so that opportunities for the disposal of food and other similar subterfuges are reduced. An adequate diet and attractive menu should be available for the patient, who should be supervised by staff during meals and for up to one hour after to reduce the possibility of self-induced vomiting. In some units, additional calories are provided by liquid supplements, for example the 'Russell Regime' a liquid diet consisting of measured amounts of Complan, Prosperol and glucose or lactose made up in 2,000 ml of fluid and given in small amounts at regular intervals throughout the day. This may be recognised as 'medicine' by the patient and, being liquid, it is not as readily disposed of as food. The calorie equivalent of this diet can be controlled by including greater or lesser amounts of the constituents and flavouring may be varied according to the patient's palate. Iron and vitamin supplements will be required unless the patient has an additional intake of solid food.

Gastro-intestinal complications may occur if re-feeding is commenced too vigorously; for example, perforation of the upper intestine, dilation of the stomach and intussusception (a telescoping of part of the small bowel) have all been recorded, so that it is usual to start with an intake of 1,000–1,500 calories per day increasing to 3,000 or 4,000 calories during the first two to three weeks of treatment. Weight gain of one kilo per week can be regarded as satisfactory, although this is often surpassed.

Formerly, modified insulin was used to improve appetite but this has not been shown to be an advantage.

Chlorpromazine, a member of the phenothiazine groups of drugs (see Chapter 18) has been used in the management of anorexia nervosa, the theory being that it reduces the resistance to eating and may possibly stimulate appetite. As the patient puts on weight, preoccupation with body image disturbance can be a distressing symptom and chlorpromazine may be useful at this stage. Some authors have advocated the use of very large doses of chlorpromazine, but hypotensive symptoms (see Chapter 18) may create problems when high doses are used and doses in excess of 150–200 mg daily may not be tolerated. Depressive symptoms may be present during treatment, but it has been stated that antidepressant drugs (see Chapter 18) are of limited value, until weight gain is satisfactory. Occasionally, electro-convulsive therapy (E.C.T.) has been used, but this is an exceptional measure.

As the target weight, that appropriate to the patients height, is approached, restrictions can gradually be lifted. (Target weight is calculated from the use of the Growth and Development charts of Dr. J. M. Tanner or similar tables.) The patient is allowed up for increasing periods of time and dietary supplements are gradually withdrawn. Sometimes the treatment regime is formalised by a specific reward schedule related to weight gain (*see* Behaviour Therapy in Chapter 19).

The role of the nurse is crucial and, especially in the early stages of treatment, a firm but understanding approach is required. Experienced nurses develop practical 'dodges' such as the use of a large plate so that an average helping of food does not appear as overwhelming as when served on a small plate. They also become very practised in recognising when the patient is somehow reneging on treatment and can subtly alter their attitudes to deal with this.

The achievement of satisfactory weight with this type of regime is not usually a problem. Difficulties arise later in helping the patient to maintain the desired weight. It is at this stage that psychotherapy, focussing on helping the patient to understand and come to terms with the emotional demands of adolescence (as outlined in Chapter 2), may be beneficial.

In a family where a member is suffering from this condition, it is distressing to see the affected person unable (or, it may appear to the family, unwilling) to eat, and it is difficult for family members not to become over-concerned in exhorting the patient to eat. It is usually easier for all concerned if they can avoid becoming involved in the eating problem and leave this to the doctor treating the patient, and to the patient herself, but in some families, gentle parental guidance may keep the situation in check.

When the patient is gaining weight, she may develop a certain degree of facial plumpness related to fluid retention. This may appear almost grotesque, but gradually weight is redistributed more naturally over the body. It is important to be aware that a patient's appearance will cause comment in the initial re-feeding stage and to help the patient understand it, rather than over-react to it. Parents should also be informed of this to anticipate the alteration in appearance so that tactless remarks can be avoided.

COURSE OF THE CONDITION

The course of anorexia nervosa varies from a single episode which responds to treatment, to a chronic disorder necessitating repeated admissions to hospital. Menstruation is rarely re-established until satisfactory weight-gain is achieved and amenorrhoea may persist for up to two years after the weight is stabilised. It may give reassurance to discuss this with the patient who is often concerned about the amenorrhoea. There are reports in the literature of patients who recover, marry and are fertile, and again, at an appropriate stage of treatment, this information may be helpful to the individual patient who has developed a fear of having become sterile.

Re-establishment of menstruation by the use of hormones has been tried. Usually it is advisable to consider this form of treatment only at the instigation of the patient, as the precipitate use of hormones by the attending physician may result in serious emotional repercussions if menstruation is unacceptable to the patient.

In the era before anti-tuberculous drugs were available, pulmonary tuberculosis contributed to the not inconsiderable mortality of this condition. In contrast, these patients rarely succumb to viral infections. There is still a mortality associated with anorexia nervosa of the order of 1 to 2 per cent, chiefly due to emaciation and death is particularly likely when the patient has lost more than 50 per cent of her body weight. Death from suicide may also occur and, at a later stage, personality problems may predominate and drug abuse can occur.

This has been a somewhat simplified account of available knowledge of anorexia nervosa, but readers interested in biochemical and other studies of the disorder may like to read further from the references given here.

REFERENCES AND FURTHER READING

*Crisp, A. H. British Journal of Hospital Medicine, 1967, 1–713.
*Dally, P. Anorexia Nervosa. Heinemann, 1969.
King, A. 'Primary and Secondary Anorexia Nervosa Syndromes.' British Journal of Psychiatry, 1963, 109–470.
Pheander, F. Act. Psych. Scan. Supplement, 24, 1970.
Russell, G. F. M. Modern Trends in Psychological Medicine. (2) Chapter 6, Page 131. Ed. J. Harding Price. Butterworth, 1970.

* Recommended selected reading

15 Sexual problems in adolescence

Before considering the sexual problems which may present in adolescence, it is important to have an understanding of the development of normal sexual behaviour. In our society a mature heterosexual relationship is regarded as the norm and where a teenager deviates from this pattern he may experience considerable distress and yet be too embarrassed to seek help. In the development of sexual behaviour there are two important areas which require consideration:

1. Biological.
2. Psychological.

BIOLOGICAL FACTORS

As soon as the child is born one of the mother's first questions relates to its sex. Is it a boy or a girl? The answer to this question is based on an examination of the external genitalia and can be given, in the majority of cases, with immediate confidence. However, there are rare abnormalities of the external genitalia which may make it difficult to reach a decision about a child's sex. Cases have been recorded where the wrong sex has been assigned at birth and, for example, a male child has been brought up as a girl only to realise later that an error has been made. At one time, it was considered that the sex could not be successfully changed after the age of three because of learned emotional attitudes, but recently cases have been described in which corrective surgery has been undertaken up to the early twenties and even then a satisfactory outcome has been achieved. In these instances, it appears that the overall emotional security of the individual and the support given by the family are at least as important as biological factors.

One particular abnormality of the penis known as hypospadias may result in a child being assigned to the wrong sex, and thereafter being brought up as a girl when in reality he is a male. On the other hand, many boys with this particular abnormality find it difficult to urinate in the erect position and in some instances boys have pleaded to be allowed to change their sex to female so that they may be less embarrassed when using the toilet at school or in other public places.

In Chapter 2, the nature of the sex organs (the ovary in the female and the testis in the male) and the hormonal secretion in

TABLE 4
Chromosomal constitution of the sexes

Sex	Male	Female
Chromosomal	XY	XX
Gonadal (primary sex organ or internal sex)	Testis producing sperm	Ovary producing ova
Hormonal	Androgens	Oestrogens
Apparent sex (external genitalia)	Penis and scrotum	Vulva

each sex was discussed, as was the chromosomal constitution of the male (XY) and of the female (XX). Table 4 is a brief reminder of the latter.

Sex chromosomal abnormalities have been reported and cases of abnormal sexual behaviour have occurred in some such individuals. For example, one girl seen by the author had an abnormal sex chromosome pattern and had felt all her life that she would like to be a boy. At the age of five she thought that her booster polio injection would turn her into a boy, she had great difficulty in coping with her obvious female development at puberty, and in keeping her aggressive behaviour in check.

Despite the complexity of the structure of the external genitalia and the abnormalities which may occur in gonadal sex, hormonal sex and chromosomal sex, biological factors seem to play quite a small part in sexual identification and it is psychological factors which are particularly important in deciding the ultimate sense of maleness or femaleness which the individual possesses. Let us therefore now consider some of these.

PSYCHOLOGICAL FACTORS

The assigned sex of an individual relates to the child's 'identification'—that is how it sees itself, as a boy or as a girl. The child's capability of attaining the standards associated with his or her assigned sex in the culture in which he or she is growing up makes a major contribution to normal psycho-sexual development. In our society, certain features are associated with each sex. Males, on the whole, are encouraged to stand up for themselves and to show a reasonable amount of aggression, whereas the tomboyish girl may be frowned on. A boy is given toy guns and tanks and plays soldiers, whereas girls are given dolls and prams and tend to play at home-making. In recent decades in our society, a prudish attitude to sex is being replaced by a more permissive approach. Many first-born children become aware of the younger brother or sister growing 'in Mummy's tummy', they see siblings being breast-fed and their questions are being answered with increasing frankness. Sex education is being undertaken in many schools and ideally, this is done before puberty. Many teenagers find it embarrassing to talk about their sexual feelings at puberty, when emotions may be titillated and self-control may be low. The question of sex education in schools remains controversial, but it does seem as though a great many children must be absent from school when sex education lessons are being given, as too many children still enter adolescence poorly informed on sexual matters! Earlier in this century, when sex was a taboo subject, teenagers were expected to control their sexual behaviour and they knew that an extra-marital pregnancy was unlikely to be tolerated within the family. But with increasing permissiveness and disparity of standards between the older generation and his own, it is often difficult for the teenager to sort out his own views. The advent of increasingly effective contraception and the recent change in the law relating to abortion has added further to the teenager's dilemma. The 'square' views of parent and teachers do little to help the developing youngster, although they may sometimes have a certain usefulness in acting as a sounding board.

Knowledge of normal sexual behaviour in contemporary British society is available as a result of a well-documented study of sexual behaviour in boys and girls aged from 15 to 19, carried out under the supervision of Michael Schofield. His study shows that by the age of 15 most boys have taken a girl out on a date. The situation is similar for girls although they in general will have started dating a year or two before boys. In the sample interviewed, twice as many boys as girls had had sexual intercourse, that is 21 per cent of the boys and 11 per cent of the girls. Dr. Schofield describes five stages of sexual activity which are useful as a guide when taking a sexual history from teenagers in order to judge which stage of maturity a particular individual has reached:

1. Little or no contact with the opposite sex: may have been taken out on a date but has never been kissed.
2. Limited experience of sexual activities: may have experienced kissing, may have experienced breast stimulation over clothes but never under clothes.
3. Sexual intimacies which fall short of sexual intercourse, experience of breast stimulation under clothes and may have experienced genital stimulation or genital apposition but no experience of sexual intercourse.
4. Sexual intercourse with only one partner.
5. Sexual intercourse with more than one partner.

With increasing age, there was a tendency for teenagers to score progressively higher on this scale and by the age of seventeen, about one-quarter of all boys had experienced sexual intercourse, though again only half that number of girls were sexually experienced. By nineteen, one-third of the boys and a quarter of the girls were sexually experienced. In the majority of cases a teenager's first experience of sexual intercourse had been unplanned. Interestingly, this first experience occurred in the home of one or other of the teenagers in more than half of the cases. Parents who are genuinely concerned about the sexual behaviour of their young people might well think twice before leaving their home to their teenage offspring. About two-thirds of the girls had had their first sexual experience with an older partner, aged twenty-one or over, the same applied to about one-third of the boys.

It appears that for many adolescents, both boys and girls, curiosity was a major factor in their first sexual experience. For the remainder, replies tended to run to type; that is, the boys said they were impelled by their sex drive whereas the girls stated that they were in love. In only a few cases did drugs appear to be a contributory factor.

In the course of the study, it appeared that promiscuity was not an outstanding feature of the usual pattern of teenage sexual behaviour. Variations of behaviour from one social group to another were noted, youngsters at secondary modern schools tending to date earlier and smoke earlier than those at grammar schools.

CONTRACEPTION

Dr. Schofield examined the question of illegitimacy and found that, as is so often the case, sexual intercourse was not premeditated and contraceptives were rarely used. Where they were used, the girl tended to rely on the boy to produce a sheath or else to 'withdraw' (*coitus interruptus*). Many girls felt that if they became pregnant, they would not wish to have the baby adopted, or have an abortion, but hoped that the boy would marry them. The boys usually realised that this was the girl's expectation and this is confirmed by the number of 'shot-gun' teenage marriages.

Professional workers with adolescents need to know about local arrangements for family planning facilities and should familiarise themselves with available contraceptive measures, for example the 'Pill' and the 'coil' for girls and the 'sheath' for men. It is important to recognise that the decision to use some form of contraception is not taken lightly by the majority of teenagers. Many girls feel that if they go on the Pill, in case their boy-friend should ask them to 'go to bed', they are acting brazenly, and others feel that, whilst they would be happier on the Pill, this would go against the standards prevailing in the parental home and their parents would be distressed if the situation came to light. So they do not take precautions and run the risk of pregnancy, rather than exposing themselves to parental displeasure.

The use of family planning services also presents problems. If the teenager is to go to a clinic which is specifically for family planning, there is always a risk that there will be someone there who will recognise her. If she goes instead to the general practitioner and he is also the family's doctor, she becomes worried in case he will divulge information to parents, either deliberately or accidentally. Sometimes a member of the family may coincidentally appear in the doctor's waiting room and enquire what is wrong with the teenager, a question which she is too embarrassed to answer. So, the teenager who should have contraceptive advice and help should be directed to a service which solves, rather than accentuates, her problems.

TERMINATION OF PREGNANCY

Of all pregnancies, it is considered that about three-quarters are carried to full-term, while one-quarter terminate prematurely; of those which terminate prematurely, somewhere between 1 in 9 and 1 in 11 will have been ended deliberately by abortion. Little more than 1 per cent of 15-year old girls at risk become pregnant, *i.e.* between 12 and 12·5 per thousand, but of these nearly two-thirds will obtain an abortion, so that less than one-third give birth to a live child.

In the 16 to 19 age group, around 8 per cent become pregnant and, of these, some 6 to 16 per cent will have an abortion. These figures are not so different from the adult rate of about 10 per cent and figures can only be approximate, as it is known that some foreigners come to this country specially to seek an abortion. It is no easy decision to decide whether a teenager merits a termination of pregnancy. Many adolescent girls request it only at their parents' instigation, often after considerable coercion and the effects of abortion in this emotionally vulnerable age group have not been adequately studied. Teenagers often consult private services to obtain an abortion and there has been little psychiatric follow-up on these patients. In the author's limited experience, it is those youngsters who have had a termination arranged privately who have usually presented with emotional symptoms, rather than those who have had a termination under the National Health Service. However, it is likely that a proportion of those terminated under the National Health Service will have been referred to the gynaecologist by a psychiatrist and will continue to receive psychiatric treatment after the pregnancy has been brought to an end.

UNMARRIED MOTHERS

On finding herself pregnant, a teenage girl may well seek a termination of pregnancy and since the passage of the 1967 Abortion Act in this country, fewer extra-marital teenage pregnancies are continuing to term. Alternatively, a teenage girl may marry the child's father and many teenage brides are pregnant at marriage. Another group of pregnant teenagers, however, decides to continue the pregnancy alone. In general, unmarried mothers of child-bearing years have been studied as groups and there have been very few attempts to examine the problems of individual pregnant adolescents. Leontine Young, in her book *Out of Wedlock*, specifically excluded those girls under the age of eighteen, but Sylvia Weir, examining a sample of unmarried mothers and their children in Scotland, picked out a group of 91 teenagers and compared them with the English teenagers in Schofield's survey, to which reference has already been made. She found that there was a general tendency for the Scottish pregnant teenager to resemble her English counterpart and for both to be relatively sexually inexperienced. This is in keeping with Anderson's comments, that Manchester teenagers conceiving extra-maritally, did so mostly as a result of the pursuit of normal adolescent activities. Weir noted that there was a higher incidence of broken homes (either by death or separation of the parents) amongst pregnant teenagers in her sample than in Schofield's sample. She found little evidence of promiscuity, but accepted that she had to rely on the teenager's accounts of their relationship with the male, which was normally described as an increasingly intimate one.

Where a teenager has decided to continue with her pregnancy, the question of the future of the unborn child must arise. Nowadays it is becoming increasingly common for teenagers to keep their children if they have the support of their own family. This may be a satisfactory solution, but many young teenagers find that it is a tremendous struggle to bring up a child on their own. Other teenagers arrange for their child to be taken into care until they are in a position to support it, or are able to provide a home when they eventually marry someone (who may not be the father of this child). Adoption is another possibility and there is some evidence to suggest that the better-adjusted teenagers tend to place their babies for adoption, while it is the immature, poorly-adjusted teenager who keeps her infant. Similarly, the better-educated mothers tend to part with their infants and the less well-educated hold on to them. As a result of such bias, all follow-up studies comparing adopted children with children who grow up with their unmarried mother, or those who are 'granny reared', must be interpreted with caution.

DEVIANT SEXUAL BEHAVIOUR

Before starting on a heterosexual relationship there may be a certain amount of rather polymorphous sexual experimentation. It would be wrong to label teenagers as transvestites, fetishists or homosexuals during what may be only a transient phase. However, for descriptive purposes, it is useful to look at different forms of sexual experimentation which may present for assessment at an adolescent clinic. For this I will use the terms which describe adult sexually deviant behaviour, but which cannot really be justifiably used in adolescence, when the patterns of sexual gratification are imperfectly established. Dr. Peter Scott has classified sexual deviation into three categories:

1. Not requiring a human partner.
2. Not requiring a willing partner.
3. Requiring a willing partner.

1. Sexual practice not requiring a human partner

a. *Fetishism**

This is a condition where sexual gratification is found in objects

* In this chapter indicates that at least one patient has presented himself with this form of sexual behaviour in a sample of 1,000 adolescents seen at an out-patient clinic over a 5-year period.

rather than people. These objects are usually related to the human body and are often associated with the opposite sex, for example, hair, underwear, shoes, gloves, or leather objects. This is a male pre-occupation. It has been suggested that the future fetishist becomes sensitised during childhood by erotic stimulation when in contact with the object. Cases of this particular problem may come to attention when a teenager is taken before a Juvenile Court charged with theft, for example of ladies' underwear taken from a neighbour's clothes line.

b. *Bestiality**
This involves the use of animals for sexual gratification. It is said to be practised by males in rural areas and very occasionally by females. Those practising bestiality may find it difficult to socialise and thus to find a human partner. Bestiality often occurs in those of lower intelligence, but this is not always the case.

c. *Transvestism**
In this condition sexual pleasure is derived from dressing in clothing of the opposite sex (cross-dressing), and most commonly the cross-dresser is a male who, after dressing in female clothing, masturbates, sometimes in front of a mirror. The clothing used is similar to the objects of the fetishist and female underclothing may be worn under male outer garments. A proportion of transvestites show an interest in wearing clothes of the opposite sex in early childhood, even as early as five to six years old, but it is usually not regarded as serious at this age. However, systematic follow-up of such young children into adult life might be both interesting and informative.

d. *Trans-sexualism**
This is a desire to change sex. It presents occasionally in children: when it occurs in adolescence one must always consider the possible onset of schizophrenia, which is sometimes accompanied by great confusion over the individual's sexual identity.

e. *Sexual asphyxia**
In this, sexual excitement is heightened when there is an element of asphyxia (that is, lack of oxygen) which may be obtained by the use

of a neck ligature, a plastic bag pulled over the head, or experimentation with anaesthetic gases. Sexual asphyxia may be associated with other deviations, for example, transvestism. Sometimes death results from sexual asphyxia, but this is usually accidental and the number of fatalities cannot be recorded accurately. It is likely that many individuals use an element of asphyxia to enhance their sexual pleasure without this coming to the attention of parents, or figures in authority. According to the late Dr. Britten, typically, when a death occurs, a man or boy is found hanged; the body is tied up with ropes, often in a complicated fashion, and usually partially undressed, naked, or partly or entirely dressed in female clothing. Experimentation may take place in a bedroom, a hut, or in an isolated wood. Murder or suicide may be suspected initially, but a clue to the sexual nature is often found, such as pornographic literature in the vicinity, and it seems that death is an accidental by-product of the deviant behaviour.

Sometimes, a nude teenager is found hanging, but unharmed, from a tree. The publicity given to such an offence is most distressing to the lad concerned. The common age range is from twelve to seventeen years of age.

2. Sexual activities not requiring a willing partner

a. Voyeurism*
In voyeurism, gratification is obtained by watching other people or animals engaged in sexual activities. For many teenagers this is a phase and such curiosity goes unrecognised. It rarely presents as a major problem, but sometimes adolescent 'peeping Toms' may be reported to the police if they have been causing annoyance.

b. Exhibitionism*
Exhibitionism is the commonest form of deviant sexual behaviour. This term is used to describe males who commit the act of indecent exposure (exposing their genitals) publicly, the indecent exposure being an end in itself and not a prelude to sexual intercourse or assault. Exhibitionism was first recognised as an offence under the Vagrancy Act of 1824, which provides that every person 'wilfully, openly, lewdly and obscenely exposing his person with intent to insult any female is a rogue and a vagabond'. It was Lasègue, in

1877, who first brought exhibitionism to medical prominence. He described the condition as occurring in men who have a sudden urge to expose their genitals, making little effort to avoid capture, often exposing themselves at the same place and the same time of day in front of the same individual. The offender may have an erect or flaccid penis and the act of exposure may be followed by masturbation. The behaviour is often inexplicable to the exhibitionist himself.

Many exhibitionists expose to young girls and it is important that the teenager should be made aware of the likelihood of encountering such behaviour. Otherwise, many may be too embarrassed or distressed to discuss the episode. Despite the commonness of this form of sexual deviation, relatively few studies are available, but one from Toronto suggests that there are two peak ages for the onset of exhibitionism—the early teens and the mid-twenties. In this Canadian study, the commonest age of onset was fifteen years and the mean age just over nineteen years.

As with other series, it was found in Toronto that many convicted offenders had a good prognosis in that they never re-appear in Court. However, the prognosis is not so good following a second Court appearance. It may be that the anxiety and publicity of the Court appearance are sufficient to help many individuals to gain control of their exhibitionistic urges subsequently, or alternatively, to become more careful in order to avoid discovery. Often teenage exposers appear to be inhibited youths who are unable to struggle against an urge to expose, although guilty and humiliated by their behaviour afterwards; there also appears to be another form involving an extroverted group of youths, who are less ashamed of their exhibitionistic urges. These latter individuals manifest other types of sexually deviant behaviour and, later, they frequently become involved in sexually violent behaviour.

Information about the family background of exhibitionists is sparse. In the Canadian study, many of the exhibitionists had a clear preference for their mothers and did not have a particularly good relationship with their fathers. It has been suggested that paternal inadequacy may be an important background factor in the development of exhibitionism; a particularly prudish background has also been commented on. Should this latter factor be so, the improvement of sex education in schools should be an important ameliorating factor. Physically, the exhibitionist's development is normal although he often presents as a rather immature individual with difficulty in sexual functioning. Probably the observer has an impression of a rather passive under-achieving individual, who is almost afraid to attempt to form a heterosexual relationship.

Exhibitionism is often an appeal for help, but unfortunately, as yet no specific treatment is available, although hormone therapy, psychotherapy (both individual and group), and behaviour therapy have all been tried. The removal of the offender to an all-male institution such as a community home of the former approved school type or Borstal, is not to his advantage, since it merely increases his difficulties in making heterosexual contacts on his return to the community.

3. Sexual activities requiring a willing partner

a. Homosexuality*
Perhaps the commonest form of sexual deviation associated with a willing partner is homosexuality. The prefix 'homo' is Greek meaning the 'same as' so that homosexuality refers to sexual activity occurring between those of the same sex. It may occur in males or females. In females it is also sometimes called lesbianism, derived from the island of Lesbos, where lived the homosexual poetess Sappho. Active homosexual relationships between women are probably less common than those between men. As discussed in Chapter 2, some adolescents pass through a period of homosexual arousal in their psycho-sexual development. This is particularly likely to occur with boys living in closed communities, as for example boarding-schools, or community homes. Younger boys may be introduced to homosexual activities by older boys. The majority of teenagers pass through the stage of homosexual experimentation to one of heterosexual arousal, but many teenagers become particularly anxious at the homosexual stage as they fear that they may be permanently homosexual. This is especially acute for those youngsters who become the butt of homosexual jokes from other teenagers. They have an awareness of their homosexual leanings at an intellectual level, although usually they have never had any homosexual experience, on account of the pressures of society against homosexuality. They may be reluctant to discuss

their problem with anyone and they become increasingly dejected
and occasionally this may be the background to a suicidal attempt.
One of the difficulties encountered by the psychiatrist treating
adolescents is in deciding which teenagers are passing through a
transient homosexual phase and which, in fact, are likely to remain
exclusively homosexual in later life. Although quite a number of
studies of male homosexuality have been published, we have as yet
difficulty in identifying the future homosexual, although some are
self-evident from an early age.

It seems that in the background of homosexuality genetic factors
are important. It has been demonstrated that in monozygotic twins
(twins arising from a single ovum) if one twin is homosexual there
is a much greater likelihood of the second twin being homosexual,
where compared with dizygotic twins (twins developing from two
ova). How these genetic factors operate is unknown.

Some workers have suggested that endocrine factors may be
important, but it is generally accepted that, whilst hormones may
influence the strength of the sexual drive, they are less likely to influence the object choice, which in general is associated with environmental factors. Therefore, it would appear that it is once more
not the seed or soil alone, but a combination of heredity and upbringing which contribute to the individual's sexual identification.
Details of the home background and its influence on the established
homosexual suggest he has often had an unsatisfactory relationship
with his father or father-figure and some would add that the situation has been further aggravated by an abnormal relationship with
the mother, especially where this has been particularly intimate. A
prudish, puritanical home background, where sexual matters are
not discussed or where they may be associated with feelings of
guilt, can also contribute to homosexual identification.

The male homosexual is frequently classified as passive or active,
according to the predominant role adopted in the homosexual
relationship. An active male homosexual tends to seek out a
relationship with another male, whereas the passive partner is
expected to submit to homosexual activity. It has been said that the
passive homosexual males are more likely to have a feminine
physique than the active male. On the other hand, an adolescent
may be a passive, or even facultative (*i.e.* functioning in either
role), homosexual when no other sexual outlet is available,

monetary gain being at least as important at times as sexual gratification. Some homosexuals may show evidence of personality impairment, being rather inadequate. In our culture, in heterosexual relationships the male is usually accepted as the dominant partner. For some passive individuals, this role may be too demanding and so passive homosexual behaviour is more acceptable. Some people have considerable anxiety about heterosexual relationships, particularly those from the sort of prudish families referred to above. Lack of confidence in his ability to make a heterosexual relationship may encourage a man to gravitate to homosexuality as an easier alternative. This is sometimes known as 'feminophobia'.

Should homosexuality be treated? The pressures of our society and the taboos against homosexuality persist, despite the change in public attitudes following recent legislation, but it is generally accepted that no attempt should be made to treat a patient for homosexuality unless it is his expressed desire. Occasionally, where Court action has supervened, the patient may wish for help so that he can become re-established in the community. In such cases the motivation of the individual patient for treatment may be difficult to establish. Various types of specialised treatment are in use, including psychotherapy, hypnosis or behaviour therapy, this last taking the form of aversion therapy, or de-sensitisation, according to the case. The response to treatment often depends on the presence of some modicum of heterosexual interest. In assessment, the Kinsey rating-scale is often used. This scale ranges from complete homosexual interest at one end, to heterosexual interest at the other. Where treatment is carried out, one would hope for a shift towards heterosexual inclinations, as indicated by the scale. In those cases where adoption of homosexual behaviour patterns is largely dictated by fear of the opposite sex, discussion of this particular barrier may be at least as helpful as behaviour therapy.

b. *Incest**

Incest can be defined as sexual behaviour occurring between persons so closely related that marriage is prohibited by law. To a certain extent therefore, it has a legal connotation. In our society, as in many others, incest is socially unacceptable and when a father is given a prison sentence on account of an incestuous relationship with his daughter, he is liable to be ostracised, if not actually attacked, by his fellow prisoners, who regard this particular crime as despicable.

Incest is usually classified into three groups:

i. Sexual relationships between a parent and child, for example father and daughter or mother and son.
ii. Sexual relationships between brothers and sisters.
iii. Sexual relationships between other blood relatives, for example uncle and niece.

In general, it would appear that father/daughter incest is much more common than mother/son incest. However, despite the data presented in the Kinsey report on sexual behaviour, there is little knowledge of the extent of incestuous sexual relationships in this country. Understandably, observations have tended to be made on selected populations, for example psychiatric patients in Northern Ireland as described by Lukianowicz, or Bagley's observations on 82 cases from psychiatric and prison sources. Analysing these 82 cases and a few additional isolated cases reported in the English literature, Bagley decided that there was no single cause of incest but that in fact he could discern at least five sub-groups.

Likewise there is little evidence of the effect of incestuous relationships on either partner. An interesting observation, confirmed by Lukianowicz, is the frequent acceptance of the situation by the mother in cases of father/daughter incest, where she certainly condones or even encourages the behaviour.

Victims of sexual offences

Another form of sexual deviation is paedophilia* where a man is sexually attracted to a young child who may be of the same or opposite sex, and in extreme cases, the end result may be sexual murder of the child. Society is much less tolerant towards the paedophiliac than to almost any other sexual deviant, usually demanding retribution and, unfortunately, the child victim may become involved in undesirable publicity and Court appearances. In a small community, it is difficult to preserve anonymity for the child. Many children who have been sexually assaulted have a period of acute distress, which, with time, becomes little more than an unpleasant memory. However, where the child has to appear in Court and again face the sexual offender, considerable further distress may result. Clearly, therefore, the child should make a statement to an experienced police officer, be medically examined and from then on, as far as possible, be excluded from subsequent events. It should be carefully explained to the parents that initially the child should have an opportunity to express his or her fears and anxieties over the assault. Thereafter the matter should not be raised again unless the child indicates a wish to discuss it. Well-meaning parents and adults may keep referring to the episode, and over-dramatise the situation. If this happens, the scar which ought to be allowed to heal can easily become a running sore.

* * *

It is difficult to put any accurate figure on the number of teenagers presenting with sexually deviant behaviour. There is no doubt, however, about the degree of distress which such behaviour causes to the individual teenager and his family. Of necessity, the various forms of sexual deviation have been described briefly here but the reader is referred to the appended list of references for further study.

REFERENCES AND FURTHER READING

Normal sexual development
*Pomeroy, W. E. *Boys and Sex*. Pelican Books 1970.
*Pomeroy, W. E. *Girls and Sex*. Pelican Books 1971.
*Rutter, M. 'Normal Psycho-Sexual Development.' Journal Child Psychol. Psychiat., 1971, *11*, 259.
*Schofield, M. *Sexual Behaviour of Young People*. Longmans, 1965. Penguin, 1968.

Unmarried mothers
Anderson, E. W. 'A Study of Extra-marital Conception in Adolescence.' Psychiat. Neurol. Basel., 1960, *139*, 313.
Barglow, P. and Bornstein, M. 'Psychiatric Aspects of Illegitimate Pregnancy in Early Adolescence.' Am. J. Orthopsych., 1968, *38*, 672.
Crellin, E., Kellmer Pringle, M. A. and Roth, T. *Born Illegitimate. Social and Educational Implications*. National Foundation for Educational Research in E. & W. 1971.

* *Recommended selected reading*

Rosen, E. J., Campbell, C. and Arime, L. 'A Psychiatric, Social and Psychological Study of Illegitimate Pregnancy in Girls under the age of 16 years.' Psychiat. Neurol. Basel., 1961, *142*, 44.

*Weir, S. *A Study of Unmarried Mothers and their Children in Scotland.* Scottish Health Further Studies. No. 13. Scottish Home and Health Dept. 1970.

Wimperis, V. *The Unmarried Mother and her Child.* Allen and Unwin, London 1960.

Young, L. *Out of Wedlock.* McGraw-Hill Book Co. Inc., New York 1954.

Sexual deviation

Bagley, C. 'The Varieties of Incest' New Society, 1st August 1969, p. 280.

Bancroft, J. H. J. 'Homosexuality in the Male.' Brit. J. Hosp. Med., 1970, *3*, 168.

Britten, R. P. 'The Sexual Asphyxias' in Gradwohl's *Legal Medicine*, Ch. 35, p. 549. Edited F. E. Camps. 2nd Edition 1968.

Kenyon, F. E. 'Homosexuality in the Female.' Brit. J. Hosp. Med., 1970, *3*, 183.

Lukianowicz, N. 'Incest.' Brit. J. Psych., 1970, *120*, 301.

Randall, J. 'Transvestism and Trans-sexualism.' Brit. J. Hosp. Med., 1970, *3*, 2, 11.

Rooth, F. G. 'Indecent Exposure and Exhibitionism.' Brit. J. Hosp. Med., 1971, *5*, 521.

*Storr, A. *Sexual Deviation.* Pelican 1964.

West, D. J. *Homosexuality.* Pelican 1960.

---

* *Recommended selected reading.*

16 The handicapped adolescent

Health is not always valued adequately by those who enjoy it, but any disruption in good health makes an impact on the sufferer and his immediate environment. A father at work is worried if he has had to leave his wife at home in bed, or if one of the children is ill. Where once, because of disease and early death, it was commonplace to fail to rear all one's offspring, the reverse is true today. With improvement in medical care, more handicapped youngsters are surviving who would not have done so in the past and they may well have a residual handicap; physical management of the handicap is outside the scope of this work, but many youngsters with long-standing physical and mental disorders do have emotional problems. In this chapter it is proposed to look at the emotional problems encountered by teenagers with:

1. Physical handicap.
2. Mental handicap.
3. Social handicap.

PHYSICAL HANDICAP

The Isle of Wight survey (Rutter, Tizard and Whitmore) showed that children with physical illness were significantly more disturbed than children in the general population, when rated on standardised questionnaires by both parents and teachers, although the form of the psychiatric disturbance (be it emotional or anti-social) associated with physical ill-health, did not differ in kind from that in the general population. Despite these observations, it must be emphasised that the majority of children with physical disorders showed no psychiatric disorder.

By the time a disabled child reaches adolescence, he is likely to have learnt to live with his handicap, but for some youngsters the additional demands of adolescence are more than they can cope with and they present with anxieties about becoming independent, their capacity to gain employment or their ability to find a life-partner. Today, with the improved facilities and special education available for some adolescents, the period of greatest stress is moving from the protected school-environment to the employment period. Blind youths, whose further training is particularly well organised, may have emotional problems, especially if training has to be at a place away from home. The strains for a sighted student moving from a small village to a college in an urban area are great, but for some of the blind they are insurmountable.

The girl born without arms may get support and encouragement even in a normal, as opposed to a special, school environment. Her achievements may not be great, but if they are reasonable and she then finds that she is virtually unemployable, this will come as a serious blow to her self-esteem and in a dejected state she may wonder about such things as her chances in the marriage-stakes. A sympathetic home environment can mean a lot to a developing youngster at this point in his or her development. Patients with chest diseases such as bronchitis or asthma, heart disease, some diabetics and epileptics, or those with orthopaedic handicaps, may find that they are unable to follow the career of their choice. A few individuals have the tenacity to overcome their handicap—Douglas Bader is a good example—but for others it is at this stage that the 'bottom falls out of their world'. So, it is necessary to consider the impact of the handicap on each individual.

Closely associated with this is the effect of the handicap on his environment, which for the more fortunate will mean a helpful family; parents may be rejecting or overprotective towards their handicapped offspring. It is often quicker for an adult to carry out an essential task, for example dressing a paralysed child handicapped as a result of polio or cerebral palsy, or carrying him, rather than waiting while he makes his way with painfully slow movements. This fosters dependence and makes adolescence with its drive towards self-reliance more difficult. Of late, in some parts of the United States of America problems such as these, and particularly those of the child who has been in hospital for a long time, have been recognised and special clubs have been formed to help such children re-integrate into the community.

To illustrate the difficulties of the handicapped young person in greater depth, it is proposed to examine the situation with reference to the epileptic adolescent. From this one may make certain generalisations concerning other disabilities.

Epilepsy

Epilepsy is one of the oldest diseases known to man. The word is derived from Greek meaning 'to take hold of' and it was referred to as the 'sacred disease' by Hippocrates.

Epileptic attacks result from a sudden abnormal electrical discharge within the brain, which may cause loss of consciousness and in some instances jerking movements of the muscle of the face, body and limbs. When these latter occur, the attack is known as a convulsion. Convulsions may occur at any age, in the new-born, in children or in adults. It is possible to induce convulsions in every individual by means of certain drugs or by passing an electrical current across the brain (see Chapter 18), but the response differs in different people and so we refer to an individual's 'convulsive threshold' which is thought to be largely genetically determined. The average individual has a relatively high convulsive threshold, so that he is unlikely to have convulsions unless a potent stimulus such as mentioned above is encountered, but in the immature child's brain, the convulsive threshold is low, so that a child with a fever associated with a high temperature may develop convulsions. These are therefore termed febrile convulsions. Where a given individual has recurring episodes of loss of consciousness due to an abnormal brain discharge, he is said to suffer from epilepsy. This is a symptom of an underlying disorder and not a disease in itself.

Two main kinds of epilepsy are recognised:

1. Generalised.
2. Focal.

Generalised epilepsy

In generalised epilepsy there is an abnormal electrical discharge across both cerebral hemispheres resulting in loss of consciousness. This loss of consciousness may be associated with a major or a minor attack.

Major attacks These are also known as *grand mal* seizures and consist of:

a. *A prodromal or warning period:* the epileptic may feel off-colour, or complain of a headache or irritability for hours or days before an attack and, if this occurs, the patient and those close to him will become aware that an attack is imminent.

b. *The fit (ictus):* The epileptic stiffens, may cry out and, if standing, will fall to the ground. His whole musculature goes into a powerful spasm, respiration ceases, the face becomes purple and the pupils dilate. After 10 to 30 seconds, jerks convulse the body, being most obvious in the face and limbs. It is these so-called *convulsive* movements which give rise to much of the fear other people experience when they see the attack. During the attack, the bladder or the bowels may be emptied. When the jerking movements cease, the muscles relax, breathing recommences and the patient resumes a normal colour. This whole phase lasts about a minute, the patient being unconscious throughout.

c. *The post-ictal phase:* With or without regaining consciousness, the patient may pass into a deep sleep; when he regains consciousness, he may show some degree of confusion, to the extent that he is unaware of his own identity or where he is. Sometimes the patient may have a headache following an attack. (Towards the end of an attack, there may be slight frothing at the mouth and the froth may be bloodstained if the patient has bitten his tongue, gums or lips.)

During a major attack it is best to leave the patient where he is, unless he is in danger from traffic, fire or other hazards. Where possible, tight clothing, particularly collars and ties, should be loosened and a wrapped pencil, spoon or handkerchief inserted between the teeth. This will prevent the patient from biting his tongue and also prevent it from falling backwards and suffocating him, but it is important not to try to *force* anything between the teeth. The patient's head should be turned to one side to discourage the tongue from falling back. The majority of epileptics need no further action to be taken during a major seizure.

Minor attacks These are another manifestation of generalised epilepsy, but are rarer. The onset of this type of attack occurs in childhood, usually before the age of fifteen. There is a characteristic abnormality of the E.E.G. (brain-wave) test known as the 'spike and wave' phenomenon. Minor seizures are notoriously difficult to control, although some of the newer anti-convulsants are helping to achieve better management of attacks. Three forms of minor attack are recognised:

a. *Petit mal* seizures or 'absences'.
b. Akinetic seizures.
c. Myoclonic seizures.

a. *Petit mal* seizures are characterised by a sudden brief loss of consciousness. The patient remains immobile and does not see or hear, being completely 'absent' from his surroundings. His gaze is fixed and his face pale. If occupied in an activity the patient will stop whatever he is doing; for example, if playing a ball game, he may just remain still for a few seconds, continuing to hold the ball. Sometimes only those nearest to the patient will be aware that anything untoward has happened. Muscle tone is diminished but is not otherwise altered, in contrast to other forms of minor attack. *Petit mal* attacks have a tendency to occur in bursts.

b. In *akinetic* seizures there is a sudden loss of muscle tone, with the result that the patient's head slumps forward and he may fall to the ground. The attack only lasts for a few seconds to that the patient, if unconscious at all, becomes conscious again almost immediately and is able to get up.

c. In *myoclonic* seizures the patient experiences sudden jerky muscle movements. Similar jerks are familiar to most people, for example when just about to drop off to sleep, but in this form of epilepsy the phenomenon is much more severe and the attack longer-lived.

Focal epilepsy
In this, an abnormal electrical discharge begins in one of the areas

of the brain and spreads to affect the whole of the brain. The clinical picture is influenced by the site of origin of the discharge and the speed of spread. If the discharge moves slowly, there may be no loss of consciousness and no convulsions, but a more rapid spread may result in unconsciousness and *grand mal* seizures. The commonest type of focal epilepsy is that known as temporal lobe epilepsy, where the site of the focus is in the temporal lobe of the brain, (*i.e.*, that part of the brain under the temple bone). In focal epilepsy, the patient may experience an aura at the beginning of the attack. This sensation lasts for seconds or, rarely, as much as a minute or more. The patient learns to recognise that this is sometimes followed immediately by loss of consciousness. The nature of the aura, such as a bright light flashing, hearing a snatch of a tune, or a smell of burning, may help in localising the affected area of the brain. Occasionally, the aura may occur without a fit and be of a type already described, or may consist of 'butterflies in the stomach' or jerking of a limb. Sometimes a patient may experience the sensation of having been in a certain situation before, (*déjà vu*) or may have a strange feeling that the world about him has changed, this latter experience being known as derealisation. Occasionally, following an attack, if the temporal lobe is involved, the patient may have a brief period of so-called 'automatic behaviour', in which he carries out more-or-less normal day-to-day activities but subsequently has no recollection of so doing.

Diagnosis
This is based on a careful history from the patient's parents and, if possible, other witnesses. Special investigations may be required in elucidating the cause of the epilepsy and making decisions with regard to drug therapy. The investigation most commonly carried out is the E.E.G. or electro-encephalogram which records the electrical activity of the brain. Small metal discs (electrodes) are stuck on the scalp, wires connect the electrodes to the recorder and, by appropriate devices, the alterations in electrical activity are recorded as waves on moving paper. The interpretation of these waves is highly skilled and special training is required to do this.

The size of the problem
About 6 to 8 school children in every 1,000 are thought to have
epilepsy, so that there are in the region of 62,000 affected school
children in the United Kingdom. Factors contributing to epilepsy
form a diverse group. There may be a genetic component, determining the level of an individual's convulsive threshold. Difficulties
associated with pregnancy and birth, particularly lack of oxygen or
a difficult delivery, may result in epilepsy. Infections of the central
nervous system, for example meningitis and encephalitis, or trauma
at birth or later (for example, a head-injury from a traffic accident)
may also be responsible. It will be appreciated that epilepsy may
occur with other handicaps and many spastic children or mentally
handicapped children may also suffer from the disorder. Autistic
children and hyperkinetic children have both been shown to
develop epilepsy in adolescence more commonly than those of
similar age in the general population.

The association between epilepsy and schizophrenia has been
commented on. For long, it was debatable whether this was a
chance association, but in 1963, Slater and his colleagues showed
that the association was greater than would arise by chance. More
recently, Taylor re-examined Slater's theories and found that the
first seizure in those patients who developed psychosis in later life
tended to occur around puberty, whereas the risk for the onset of
true epilepsy is greater in childhood.

Management
1. Anti-convulsants.
2. Education.

1. *Anti-convulsants* These are drugs which control, but do not
cure, epilepsy. The aim in their use is to reduce the frequency and
the severity of seizures. Once the decision has been taken to start
drug-therapy, it should be continued until the patient has been free
of fits for at least three years. It is usual to start the drug cautiously,
slowly increasing the dose until seizures are controlled or side
effects arise. If the patient fails to respond to the selected drug, a
second one may be substituted, again starting with a small dose
and gradually increasing. We shall consider these medications in a
little detail since it may be useful for the non-medical reader to be
aware of their usage.

The medications most commonly used in *grand mal* seizures and focal epilepsy are:

a. *Phenytoin sodium* (Epanutin) This is the most useful member of the hydrantoin group of drugs. It is less likely to cause drowsiness and depression than phenobarbitone and the dose is 50 to 100 mg two or three times a day.

b. *Phenobarbitone* This is a long-acting barbiturate which some years ago was the most commonly used anti-convulsant, but in view of the likelihood of it causing adverse effects such as depression in adults and restlessness in children (particularly those with temporal lobe seizures), it is less popular than formerly. The dose is 30 mg, two or three times a day.

c. *Primidone (Mysoline)* If a patient fails to respond to phenytoin or phenobarbitone, primidone may be added or substituted for phenobarbitone. Chemically, this drug is similar to phenobarbitone and is metabolised to phenobarbitone in the body and it is liable to cause drowsiness even on a small dose. It is customary to start with a low dose, for example, 125 mg daily increasing to a maximum of 750 mg to 1 gramme per day in divided doses.

d. *Sulthiame (Ospolot)* This drug has been found to be particularly useful in temporal lobe epilepsy, and focal epilepsy, particularly when used in association with phenytoin. The dose is 50 to 150 mg two or three times a day. The dose has to be increased gradually because of possible unwanted side effects. Recently it has been suggested that the effect of this drug is merely to increase the blood level of other anti-convulsants and that it itself has no specific anti-convulsant effect.

e. *Carbamazepine (Tegretol)* This has lately been used in the treatment of epilepsy and it has been suggested that it is of particular value when behaviour disorders are associated. The dose is 100 to 200 mg two or three times a day.

Drugs most commonly used in the treatment of minor attacks include:

a. *Ethosuximide (Zarontin)* This drug has been found to be particularly effective in the treatment of *petit mal* attacks associated with a 3-cycles per second spike-and-wave abnormality on the brain wave test and its use should probably be confined to this particular type of minor seizure, replacing the formerly used troxidone (Tridione). The dose is 250 mg two or three times daily.

b. *Sodium valproate (Epilim)* Although only recently introduced into the range of available anti-convulsants this drug is proving very useful in the control of minor seizures, including myoclonic seizures which have always been especially difficult to control. With increasing experience in its use it is likely that it will become the drug of choice in the treatment of minor seizures, including *petit mal* attacks associated with 3-cycles per second spike-and-wave phenomenon on the E.E.G. and its use in other types of attack will increase. Side effects appear to be rare, but the drug can potentiate the effect of other anti-convulsants which may then produce side effects. When this occurs the treatment is to reduce the dose of the other drugs. The dose is initially 200 mg three times a day increasing to 800 mg to 1,400 mg a day.

c. *Clonazepam (Rivotril)* This is another anti-convulsant which has become available only recently. It belongs to benzodiazepine group of drugs, a group discussed in some detail in Chapter 18. Largely used on account of their ability to reduce anxiety, it was noted that one of them, diazepam (Valium), was also beneficial in controlling convulsions and had a normalising effect on the electroencephalogram. The closely related clonazepam has now superseded diazepam in the treatment of epilepsy and is particularly valuable in the treatment of *status epilepticus*, a serious complication of epilepsy, in which the patient suffers one major attack after another and is at risk of death from exhaustion. Clonazepam is now the drug of choice in treating this emergency. Its place in the routine management of major and minor attacks has yet to be established, but the indications are that it will be a valuable anticonvulsant, especially where patients suffer from more than one type of attack. The dose is 1 or 2 mg three times daily.

Many epileptics require a combination of drugs to achieve adequate control of attacks. It is essential that additional drugs should be introduced gradually, and that the drug which is being replaced is withdrawn by a slow decrease in dose. Some drugs, notably some of the anti-depressants and the so-called major tranquillisers (*see* Chapter 18), lower the convulsive threshold and if they have to be prescribed for an epileptic it may be necessary to increase the dose of anti-convulsants given.

Table 5 summarizes the available preparation of commonly-used anti-convulsants.

2. *Education* In view of the liability to sudden loss of consciousness, patients with uncontrolled epilepsy must avoid certain potentially dangerous situations. They are discouraged from cycling, or at least cycling alone; swimming may only be undertaken if they are accompanied by a responsible person, who is aware of the patients' tendency to have epileptic attacks and undertakes to keep a close watch on them; when having a bath, they should be asked not to lock the door. In the employment situation, it is inadvisable to work with unguarded, fast-moving machinery, or to be adjacent to large stretches of open water, open electrical circuits, unguarded fires, ovens or hot plates. Working at a height if unguarded, working with fragile or valuable equipment, and certain jobs involving sole responsibility for the care of small children, all may present difficulties. When applying for a driving licence, any tendency to loss of consciousness must be declared and it is illegal for an epileptic to possess a driving licence unless fits have been completely controlled for a minimum period of three years. Apart from these provisos, the epileptic should be urged to lead as normal a life as possible. There is evidence to suggest that stimulating activities reduce the likelihood of a fit and that boredom increases the probability, so attempts should always be made to engage the epileptic in interesting and productive pursuits.

Once a diagnosis of epilepsy is made, it is important to explain the implications of this to the child and his parents, so that they are understood from the outset. Visits to a hospital specialist or family doctor involves inspection of a record of attacks and making any necessary alterations in medication but, in addition, should always allow time to discuss queries and anxieties with the child and his parents. Parents must be encouraged not to overprotect the child as this is more common than rejection in our culture, although in some immigrant populations rejection is seen. As with physical handicap, many adolescents cope with the aid of a supportive school environment but there are understandable anxieties in rela-

TABLE 5
Anti-convulsants

Official Name	Trade Name	Preparations	Usual dose
Phenobarbitone	Gardenal	15 mg, 30 mg, 60 mg, 100 mg Tablets	30 mg t.d.s.*
Phenobarbitone sodium	Gardenal sodium	200 mg per ml Injection	
Phenytoin sodium	Epanutin	50 mg, 100 mg Capsules Suspension 30 mg per 5 ml Injection 50 mg in 1 ml	50 mg–100 mg b.d.* or t.d.s.
Primidone	Mysoline	250 mg Tablets 250 mg per 5 ml. Suspension	125–250 mg t.d.s.
Carbamazepine	Tegretol	100 mg, 200 mg Tablets 100 mg per 5 ml Syrup	100 mg initially 200 mg t.d.s.
Sulthiame	Ospolot	200 mg, 50 mg Tablets 50 mg per 5 ml Suspension	100 mg initially with gradual increase to 1 g daily if necessary
Ethosuximide	Zarontin, Capitus or Emeside	250 mg Capsules Syrup 250 mg per 5 ml	250 mg b.d. or t.d.s.
Methsuximide	Celontin	300 mg Capsules	300 mg initially gradually increasing to 300 mg t.d.s.
Clonazepan	Rivotril	0·5 mg, 2 mg Tablets Injection 1 mg	1–2 mg t.d.s.
Diazepam	Valium	2 mg, 5 mg, 10 mg Tablets 2 mg, 5 mg Capsule Syrup 2 mg per 5 ml Injection 10 mg in 2 ml	5 mg t.d.s.
Sodium valproate	Epilim	200 mg Tablets 200 mg per 5 ml Syrup	200–400 mg t.d.s.

* b.d. = twice daily; t.d.s. = three times daily.

tion to employment and marriage. It is important to encourage as realistic an attitude to such employment as a teenager can accept, since there are some occupations from which he will be barred in his own interests and for the safety of others. Despite the lack of understanding by the general public about epilepsy, which may create difficulties in employment, it is better for an individual to be frank about his susceptibility to epileptic attacks, as concealment can increase difficulties. In some instances, frankness has helped a handicapped teenager to get a job, as the prospective employer has been impressed by his honesty, but admittedly the reverse also applies in too many cases.

Epilepsy should not be a bar to marriage. If it is a result of birth injury, accident or infection, there is no likelihood of epilepsy being passed on to the next generation. Where the cause of the disorder is not clear, the possibility of offspring being affected can be discussed by the patient with his family doctor and/or hospital specialist and in some instances genetic counselling may be desirable. Sometimes, if fits are uncontrolled, it may be necessary to postpone a family for a period as there is always the risk of dropping a baby during an attack. If it is decided to postpone starting a family for some time, it is important when seeking advice on family planning to disclose the fact that the patient is an epileptic, so that the most appropriate help may be given.

Witnessing an epileptic attack for the first time can be most distressing. This is particularly so for parents, to whom it may appear as if their child has died. Their response at this time may set the scene for the family's reaction for years to come. Some families may adopt a policy of letting the child have his own way, in case thwarting him should provoke a further attack. Unfortunately, the outcome of this policy is often that he becomes so used to having his own way that he becomes unpopular with his contemporaries and does not fit into the educational or employment scene. At this stage his social difficulties may create greater problems than his epilepsy. Similarly, in the educational situation, it should be explained to the teacher that the pupil has epilepsy, the type of fit should be described and what should be done if he has an attack, but overall the teacher ought to be encouraged to treat him as an otherwise normal child. It is relatively easy to explain to a teacher at a primary school that a child has epilepsy, but often at secondary school it may be difficult to pass on the information to all the teachers concerned. The author is aware of one instance where a class was being taken by a student teacher and an epileptic with *petit mal* was reading aloud and suddenly stopped. The student teacher was unaware of the nature of the problem, and ridiculed the pupil in front of the class, with most unfortunate results for the child.

Some epileptics have learning difficulties, on account of distractibility and limited attention span. They may listen to the teacher for a short period and then become distracted by a stimulus in the class room and 'shut-off'. By the time their thoughts return to the teacher they have missed several sentences and so may be unable to follow the remainder of the lesson. For these children it is important to be in a class where there is a good pupil/teacher ratio and the teacher must understand the nature of the difficulty, so that each child can work at his or her own pace.

There are some special schools for epileptics and, occasionally, children who have severe attacks which are difficult to control may require such education, but a majority of staff at these special schools claims that most of their pupils are there because of associated behavioural disorders, or because of family problems, rather than because of the epilepsy itself.

The British Epilepsy Association is a voluntary organisation which aims at improving the community's understanding of epilepsy and providing advice and information to epileptics, employers and any others who are intrested. In addition, it organises conferences and supports and encourages research. In many areas it also promotes social functions which are helpful to some epileptics who would otherwise be very isolated.

MENTAL HANDICAP

With the development of techniques for measuring intelligence at the turn of the century, it became possible to distinguish between mental illness and mental handicap although occasionally the two may co-exist. Previously in this country the mentally handicapped were known as 'mentally subnormal' 'mentally deficient' or 'mentally retarded'.

When tests were devised to measure intelligence, it was customary to talk about a child's 'mental age' and to compare it with his actual age; for example, a child of six years who could perform tasks which an average eight-year-old could carry out would be said to have a mental age of eight but an actual age of six. This implied that he had superior abilities for his age. Contrariwise, the child aged five who could only perform tasks done by the majority of four-year-olds would have a mental age of four years and an actual age of five years and would be less intelligent than the majority of children of his age. However the concept of mental age was somewhat clumsy so the term 'intelligence quotient' or 'I.Q.' was introduced. Initially, this was obtained by calculating the child's mental age, dividing this by his actual age and multiplying by 100, i.e.

$$\frac{\text{Mental age}}{\text{Actual age}} \times 100 = \text{I.Q.}$$

Thus, in the example given above, the bright child would have an I.Q. of $\frac{8}{6} \times 100 = 133$ and the dull child, $\frac{4}{5} \times 100 = 80$. It will be apparent that Mr. Average will have a mental age of 6 when his actual age is 6 and he will have an I.Q. of 100; in fact his I.Q. could be 99 or 101 and from statistical manipulation it is now accepted that Mr. Average has an I.Q. in the range of 90–110. About 20 per cent of the population has an I.Q. above 110, so are of superior intelligence, and another 20 per cent have an I.Q. in the 70—90 range. Those with an I.Q. below 70 are regarded as being mentally handicapped. For those who are statistically sophisticated this means that the mentally handicapped are those who, on a test which has a mean of 100 and a standard deviation of 15, score two standard deviations below the mean. About 2·5 to 3 per cent of children are so classified.

Some years ago it was customary to classify the mentally handicapped into three grades:

1. 'Idiots' with an I.Q. under 20.
2. 'Imbeciles' with an I.Q. 20–50.
3. 'Feeble minded' with an I.Q. 50–70.

This classification finds little favour as it is now recognised that it is often the child's personality traits, whether he is ambulant and whether he is continent, which are the important factors in deciding his social future rather than his I.Q. Also, the terms had come to be derogatory and emotive so they are never used nowadays.

The majority of mentally handicapped children are relatively mildly retarded, but about one in ten has severe intellectual retardation with an I.Q. of less than 50. In the majority of these children organic brain disease is the cause of the retardation and is often associated with physical disorder, whereas in the group with an I.Q. in the 50 to 70 range, although some may have organic brain pathology, genetic and social factors are more important.

Whereas in the past many mentally handicapped children were forced to grow up in institutions, with the recent emphasis on community care many more mentally retarded young people are living at home and going to school, employment or sheltered workshop. Until April 1971, the less severely handicapped (I.Q. 50 to 70) were educated in special schools for the educationally subnormal, but now in some areas there is a tendency to teach them in special classes in the neighbourhood school. The more grossly retarded (I.Q. below 50) who were previously known as the severely subnormal were regarded as ineducable, but if they were not incontinent they might attend a junior training centre run by the Health Department of the local authority. In April 1971, these training centres became the responsibility of the Education Department as it was recognised that no child should be deemed ineducable. Each child should be educated up to the level of his ability so the former training centres now form part of the special schools provision and schools in hospitals for the mentally handicapped have become the responsibility of the Local Education Authority.

The mentally-handicapped child appears to have an increased vulnerability to the types of environmental stress that create problems in all children, but they are particularly sensitive to cultural and emotional deprivation. There is some evidence to suggest that the mentally handicapped child brought up in his home environment will be more likely to develop his abilities to an adequate functional level than a similar child brought up in an institution. This is particularly true for language development. On the other hand, the presence of a mentally-handicapped child in the home can cause a considerable strain on the family's emotional resources. In their study, Tizard and Grad have described the burden of care which those families carry when a subnormal child is living with them, as opposed to the family with a subnormal child growing up in an institution. As with the physically-handicapped child, the parents may react by rejecting the child, or by being overprotective. It is often difficult enough for parents of normal children to get baby-sitters at times, but the problems are magnified for the family with a mentally-handicapped child since inexperienced people are understandably apprehensive about agreeing to look after a handicapped child in case a situation should arise with which they might be unable to cope. On the other hand, over-protective parents may be reluctant to trust their 'special' child to a baby-sitter.

Siblings of a handicapped child may resent what they see as the monopolising of parental attention. There is some truth in this, as many mentally-handicapped children have a prolonged infancy, being late in learning to walk and in gaining control of bowel and bladder. Laundry bills may strain financial resources, so that the other children feel they are being deprived of pocket-money and it is always much harder to organise things like a day's outing for the family. Sometimes, siblings may be ashamed of their mentally handicapped brother or sister, for example, a child, who took a family photograph to show to the other pupils at school, was subjected to ridicule because a brother with Down's Syndrome (mongolism) appeared in the family group. Until this incident, it had not occurred to the child to conceal the fact that he had a handicapped brother. Some teenagers may be reluctant to bring their friends home because of the presence of the handicapped sib. Apart from such problems and adjustments, in the few studies that are available there is no evidence that the presence of a handicapped child in the home usually creates any serious emotional disturbance among the healthy siblings.

As with other children, the personality of the parents, their consistency and their capacity to deal with the handicapped child's problems are of particular importance. The child's temperament is also of significance in his adaptation. If he is able to relate to others and is emotionally stable, he may be able to integrate into the lower streams of the ordinary school and present no great problem. On the other hand, behaviour disorders become increasingly common the lower down the intelligence scale one goes. In the Isle of Wight study (Rutter *et al.*) the parent and teacher questionnaires showed that behavioural psychiatric disorders are likely to occur in some 30 to 40 per cent of intellectually retarded children. On the whole their psychiatric disorders do not follow any specific pattern, the rates for neurosis, conduct disorders, personality disorders and developmental disorders being similar to, although higher than, those of the children of higher intelligence. For the retarded child, even more than for the child of average intelligence, the environment can be stressful at times. He rapidly becomes aware that he is a disappointment to his parents and he certainly cannot compensate for other deficiencies by academic achievements. He is also more liable to be rejected as a playmate by other children in the neighbourhood. And, just as he has difficulty in academic learning, he may also have difficulty in learning socially acceptable behaviour. In those cases in which an element of brain dysfunction plays a part, the development of self-control may be impaired and the child may habitually over react to situations, which can sometimes make him a difficult companion.

As mentally-handicapped children approach adolescence they experience the same biological changes and drives as those outlined in Chapter 2. They may be concerned about their abilities to obtain employment, to live independently in the world, and to have a family of their own. Many mentally-handicapped young people have less control of these drives than adolescents of average intelligence, so that 'acting out' in terms of sexual behaviour and aggression may be quite serious in a small minority. When this happens, psychotherapy at a simple level may be helpful. For these patients, the treatment is in fact similar to that discussed in the third section of this book, allowance being made for their intellectual limitations.

The parents of mentally-handicapped children living at home require much more help and support than is at present generally available, particularly during adolescence. Anxiety in the family may rise as the mentally handicapped teenager gets bigger, especially if there are any problems with violent behaviour. If parents have a healthy attitude towards the handicapped child, difficulties in adolescence are usually not great but a small group of mentally-handicapped children who have grown up in the community may require admission to hospital to help them to come to terms with their adolescent development.

The question of contraception for the handicapped adolescent is a subject with which society will have to come to terms. Certainly, parents should feel that they can discuss this with the family doctor or hospital specialist who is involved with the care of their offspring. It is not necessarily that the handicapped are more promiscuous, but self-evidently they have less knowledge and capacity for foresight than their intellectually normal peers.

Employment

Many emotionally-stable individuals with mental handicap are quite capable of undertaking jobs involving a regular, un-complicated routine and often derive great satisfaction from being able to play their part in the community. Sometimes, however, their superiors are so impressed with their standard of work that they feel it would be rewarding to move them to a rather more difficult task which would bring greater remuneration. This step may be the first one towards disaster, as the new task may be too complicated for the mentally-handicapped individual to comprehend. His per-formance may tail off, but rather than demote him to his previous job, he may be paid off and then have great difficulty in obtaining further employment. It is, therefore, not always a kindness to en-courage a mentally-handicapped person to seek promotion. The situation here is somewhat similar to that already discussed in Chapter 5 on schizophrenia.

SOCIAL HANDICAP

Adoption

This was defined in the Horsburgh report of 1937 as follows: '. . . the essence of adoption, whether legalised or *de facto*, seems to us to rely on the creation of an artificial relationship analogous to that of parent and child which is accepted by all parties as permanent. The child is absorbed into the family of the adopters and treated as if it were their own natural child.'

Adoption has been known since Biblical times. It is said that the earliest formal record of adoption is a Sumerian cuneiform tablet dated around 2360 B.C. In Hebrew literature, the most famous adoption is that of Moses. In these earlier times, adopted children had a secure legal status in their family and the birth of subsequent legitimate children did not deprive them of their rights, but in England in feudal times, the bastard of lowly origin had no legal rights.

In Tudor England, bastardy was more or less socially accepted, but with the rise of Puritanism and the introduction of the Poor

Law legislation, a social stigma again began to be attached to illegitimacy. Following the Industrial Revolution, the illegitimate child was frequently abandoned by its mother and subsequently died. It was only in the second half of the nineteenth century that there was growing concern for deprived children, epitomised by Dr. Barnardo and the London Society for the Prevention of Cruelty to Children. Gradually, a more enlightened attitude developed to illegitimacy, but it was only in 1926 that adoption was legally recognised in this country. The impetus towards adoption arose from the First World War, where the heavy loss of male life and an increased illegitimacy rate, made the community aware of the importance of child lives. Gradually, organisation developed which attempted to place the right child in the right home. Initially, placements were voluntary and many voluntary organisations continue up until the present time. Some local authority Children's Departments interpreted the 1948 Children Act as allowing them to arrange for adoptions, but it was really after the implementation of the 1958 Children Act that local authority Social Services Departments generally took the power to place children for adoption. However, with improved contraception, the passage of the Abortion Act in the 1960s, and the current trends for unmarried mothers to keep their children and bring them up in single parent families, the supply children for adoption has decreased to a marked extent.

It has been estimated that the percentage of adopted children in the population as a whole in both the United States of America and the United Kingdom is between one and two per cent. Over half are thought to be extra-familial adoptions (*i.e.*, babies who are adopted by people with whom there is no blood tie). The remainder are intra-familial adoptions and, for example, an infant may be adopted by his maternal grandparents, particularly if the mother is unmarried and is one of a sizeable family. Estimates of successful adoptions vary widely, the figures ranging from 50 to 90 per cent. Similarly, estimates of the degree of disturbance amongst adopted children show a good deal of variation. Pringle, in Great Britain, found that the prevalence of adopted children in schools for the maladjusted is 8 per cent, and in similar institutions in the United States of America it has been found to be 12 per cent, whilst amongst delinquents of good intelligence it has been shown to be 27 per cent. (However, this last figure is from special schools, which serve the higher-income groups in the United States of America.) Several reports concerning adopted children who have been referred to children's psychiatrists indicate that, proportionally, more adopted children are referred to a psychiatrist than their representation in the general population. Humphrey and Ounstead, from the Park Hospital, Oxford, reported on eighty adopted children seen in the Oxford area between January 1951 and April 1962. These were extra-familial adoptees, and two boys were referred for every girl. This hospital sample represented a frequency of 2·9 per cent of adoptees, which is twice the expected frequency of referrals from the general population. This increase in the rate of referral to a children's psychiatrist has also been found in other countries. For this and other reasons, there has been considerable research interest in adopted children over the last eighteen to twenty years and a few facts have emerged. Children adopted under the age of six months and preferably under the age of three months are less likely to run into difficulties. It is important that children growing up are made aware of their adoptive status from as early an age as possible, but particularly before they start school. The need for this was underlined in Dr. Alexina McWhinney's work entitled *Adopted Children and How They Grow Up* which is the report of a study based on interviews with adults who had been adopted in childhood. There are many striking examples in this work of how adopted children, not told, so often learnt of it at school.

Although adopted children may be referred to a psychiatrist for behavioural complaints, such as enuresis or obsessional symptoms, those adopted later in childhood are found to have a tendency towards more severe anti-social symptoms. A few of those who do not present severe psychiatric disorders may have emotional difficulties, which become particularly poignant at adolescence when they are struggling to establish their identity. The teenager growing up in an intact home may have similar difficulties, but these can be greatly magnified for the adopted child, who struggles with problems in relation to both his real and his adopted parents. Many adopted children have a rich fantasy life in relation to their real parents. They are sometimes reluctant to discuss this with their adoptive parents, in case they will hurt their feelings and even when they screw up the courage to broach the subject they find that the adoptive parents do not have sufficient knowledge of the real parents to answer the children's questions. An area of anxiety in the adopted adolescent's mind sometimes relates to heredity, in case they have inherited any undesirable characteristics.

Many adopted teenagers are anxious to meet their real parents, but for so many, the search itself is more important than actually finding their parents. Many are aware that, in reality, they might be disappointed by such an encounter. About 80 per cent of adopted children in this country are born illegitimately and adopted girls from this background sometimes have profound anxieties about their own ability to control their sexual drives. The adoptive parents may also have understandable anxieties over this, wondering if the teenager will 'end up' as her real mother did.

In an earlier chapter the importance of the environment in which the child grows up was stressed, and for adopted children the need for a stable background is paramount.

Illegitimacy
Some illegitimate children growing up in foster-homes, or children's homes, or living with unmarried mothers, have anxieties at adolescence similar to those of the illegitimate child who has been adopted. If the everyday environment cannot provide the degree of reassurance and stability these particular teenagers require, it may sometimes be necessary to recruit psychiatric help in order to allay the anxiety.

Children from broken homes
Where the home has been broken, other than by the death of a parent, the teenager may at first accept the situation and be quite content to live with the parent who has been given custody. Then suddenly he begins to examine the background to the parental separation more closely and starts to ask questions. This is particularly so where one parent does not have access and his or her shadowy figure is almost unknown to the adolescent. As with the adopted child, he may develop fantasies about the missing parent, to the distress of the parent with whom he is living and many such teenagers set out to discover the whereabouts of their missing parent. Again, as with the adopted child, the search may be more

important than finally locating the parent and, although we may inform the teenager of steps which can be taken to locate a missing
person, it is usually unwise to take the initiative but, instead, let him
or her dictate the pace. Often they spontaneously work through
their emotional feelings and in this event do not usually take active
steps to locate the parent.

Many Courts, when giving custody of a child to one parent, allow
the other parent access. In the parent's eyes this is mandatory, but
she (or more usually he) may only be free to visit the child over the
week-end. As children in this situation approach adolescence, they
want to join in activities with their own age-group and where
formerly they enjoyed afternoon treats with the parent not living at
home, may come to resent these visits. They then see the parental
visits as an intrusion on their free time and a slight to their approaching adulthood. Perceptive parents become aware of this
situation and attempt to fit in with their teenage offspring's
programme.

By adolescence, many teenagers are quite capable of deciding
which parent will make the best provision for their individual needs
and in many Courts nowadays the teenager is allowed to express an
opinion when custody is being decided upon. Legislation may improve this situation further in the future, so that the teenager's
opinion will always be taken into account.

'Uncommon statistical deviance' as a cause of emotional disturb-ance

By and large, children are conforming beings and they like to be the
same as other children. Therefore, the one who stands out from his
own age group for any reason, for example, by being excessively
short or excessively tall, exceptionally intelligent or exceptionally
dull for his environment (for example, the relatively-dull child of
academic parents), may present with emotional difficulties. Occasionally, it may be possible to bring about some form of environmental readjustment and simple discussions may also help the
child to come to terms with his problems. The child with the most
difficulty in accepting that he is different, often has other emotional
problems which may be expressed by focussing attention on his
deviation. When this occurs, psychiatric treatment in more depth
may be necessary.

REFERENCES AND FURTHER READING

Rutter, M., Tizard, J. and Whitmore, K. *Education, Health and Behaviour*. Longman, 1970.

Epilepsy

Jeavons, P. M. 'The Practical Management of Epilepsy.' Hospital Update, 1975, *1*, 11.
Pryse-Phillips, W. *Epilepsy*. John Wright and Sons. Bristol 1969.
Scott, D. *About Epilepsy*. Duckworth, London, Rev. Edtn. 1973.
Slater, E. T. O., Beard, A. W. and Glithero, E. 'The Schizophrenia-like Psychoses of Epilepsy.' Brit. J. Psychiat., 1963, *109*, 95.

Mental handicap

Adams, M. and Lovejoy, H. *The Mentally Subnormal: Social work Approaches*. Heinemann, 1972.
Heaton-Ward, W. A. *Mental Subnormality*. John Wright and Sons Ltd. 1975.
Gath, A. 'The Effect of Subnormality on the Family.' Brit. J. Hosp. Med., 1972, *8*, 147.
Tizard, J. and Grad, J. *The Mentally Handicapped and Their Families*. Maudsley Monograph No. 7. Oxford University Press. 1971.

Adoption

Humphrey, M. and Ounstead, C. *Adoptive Families Referred for Psychiatric Advice*. 1. 'The Children.' Brit. J. Psych., 1963, *109*, 599. 2. 'The Parents.' Brit. J. Psych., 1964, *110*, 549.
McWhinney, A. *Adopted Children and How They Grow Up*. Routledge and Kegan Paul. 1967.
Pringle, M. L. K. *Adoption: Facts and Fallacies*. Longmans, 1966.

PART 3
TREATMENT AND MANAGEMENT
OF THE DISTURBED ADOLESCENT

17 The first interview
and principles of treatment

Treatment commences from the moment of referral to the psychiatric clinic. The confrontation of the teenager with the fact that there is sufficient concern about his problems and/or behaviour to suggest referral to a specialist clinic initiates a chain of reaction. His first emotion may be one of relief, that at last help may be forthcoming; of anxiety, that he is considered to be going out of his mind (because the stigma of psychiatric referral persists); or of anger and hostility.

The act of referral is no indication that an appointment will be kept and failed appointments are not uncommon at adolescent clinics. We have no knowledge of the number of teenagers to whom psychiatric help is offered, but refused. The fact that an appointment is kept is often the outcome of a considerable amount of work by the referring agent before the initiation of the referral, by the family doctor, the social worker or the school teacher. It is sometimes apparent from failed appointments that there has been little or no preparation of the prospective patient. Knowledge of the clinic, its staff and its method of working may be useful, since the referring agent can impart some of this information to the teenager and thus some anxiety may be allayed at the outset.

At the diagnostic interview at the clinic similar emotions will be apparent, although often relief is tinged with anxiety. An adult patient has some idea of what to expect but for an unsophisticated teenager the journey to a strange hospital or clinic, perhaps in an unfamiliar part of the city, will be something of an ordeal in itself even if he or she is accompanied by an adult.

The receptionist has an important role to play here. She is often the first person in the hospital to meet the patient and her attitude, whether reassuring, pleasant or abrupt, can make the psychiatric interview easier or more difficult.

Many teenage patients feel that they have been coerced into coming to visit a psychiatrist and see no reason to be co-operative. Their attitude may even be apparent in the waiting room. The psychiatrist seeing an adolescent patient has often to work much harder to establish rapport than a colleague seeing children or adults. He also has to convey to the adolescent sufficient of his professional expertise for the adolescent to be able to come to a decision about accepting a further appointment; in other words, the psychiatrist has to 'sell' himself and his knowledge to the teenager at an early stage.

At the clinic, the adolescent patient will usually be accompanied by parents, a guardian and/or a professional colleague. The psychiatrist has to decide whom to see first. In most instances, it is desirable to interview the teenager first. This is particularly so if he has been referred because of anti-social problems. If the parents or professional worker have the first opportunity to give their account of the problems and background features, the teenage patient may be antagonised. If the adolescent is seen first, he feels that his point of view will be listened to, even if not wholly accepted. If he is too ill to give a clear account of his difficulties, or of too limited intelligence to give a reliable history, the interview can be terminated tactfully but fairly rapidly and no harm is done. It is also useful to see the patient and parents together at some stage.

Again, while the adult patient may have some understanding of the psychiatrist's method of working, it is likely that this will not be so for an adolescent. For example, if his problem is one of difficulty in sleeping, he may become impatient with the psychiatrist who enquires about his school or work situation. It is sometimes helpful to explain to the adolescent that in order to understand the situation properly, the psychiatrist finds it important to have an understanding of his home and educational background so that he can discover how the teenager has coped with stresses in the past. The psychiatrist then proceeds to take a detailed history covering family and home background, a history of the teenager's development, education and, if appropriate, occupation.

Usually, enquiries are also made about psycho-sexual development. The reasons why the teenager has been referred to the clinic are gone into in some depth. This can be disconcerting to someone who may only have been told a few hours previously of the appointment. If the reason for referral is stealing or some other antisocial problem, the teenager may not be prepared to discuss this with a complete stranger immediately. For this sort of reason, particularly if the referring agent has not made the problem clear, many psychiatrists find that the teenager appreciates being given the opportunity to discuss those parts of his history which are not emotionally charged before being asked to discuss the presenting problem in detail. Sensitive areas often become apparent at an early stage of the interview and in some instances it is advisable to leave further examination of such areas until a subsequent interview.

The aim of the first interview is to obtain some awareness of the problem and work out a provisional formulation with regard to diagnosis and treatment. If too much pressure is exerted on a teenager at the initial interview, a further appointment may not be kept. Alternatively he may lie about habits of which he is ashamed, particularly if there are moral overtones (for example, pre-marital sexual activity). It is difficult for a teenage patient to retract any erroneous impression that he has given to the psychiatrist, without loss of face, and so progress and treatment may be hampered because of the psychiatrist's attitude at the diagnostic interview. When a patient has been referred specifically for a Court report, however, it is important to obtain all the relevant facts at the initial interview unless a subsequent one can be fitted in before the Court appearance.

Adequate information from the referring agent is invaluable. For example, knowledge that a youngster has recently been bereaved of a parent may enable the psychiatrist to approach the family history with particular care and so avoid an unncessarily distressing interview.

Most psychiatrists working with teenagers learn to frame questions in a tactful way; for example, 'Who lives at home?' If mention is made of only one parent, brothers or sisters, one knows to make cautious enquiries about the unmentioned parent, such as 'Did you ever know your father (or mother)?' In this way the question of death, divorce, separation or illegitimacy can be approached relatively freely. A patient may be known to be adopted, but he may not be aware that this information is available to the psychiatrist and it is both instructive and desirable to wait to see at which, if any stage of the interview the teenager divulges this fact. It is obviously important to use words that the teenager can easily understand. Questions should be framed in a way which is least damaging to self-esteem. It is better to ask, 'With what school subjects do you have most difficulty?' rather than, 'What is your worst subject?'

A boy or girl who is obviously pre-pubertal may be upset if asked outright about sexual relations. It is extremely unlikely from the stage of physical development that he or she will be active in this area and inappropriate questions may suggest to the patient that the psychiatrist has some kind of 'hang-up!' For other youngsters this may be a problem area, but one which they would be too embarrassed to broach, so that careful and tactful questioning and an understanding manner is required.

Ideally, a physical examination should be carried out. For those patients who are unlikely to return for a second visit, this is done at the end of the first interview. For other patients who will have a further appointment it may be felt more appropriate to carry it out at the second visit, to reduce embarrassment and to prevent any impression of haste.

In adult psychiatry, interviewing a relative or friend of the patient, to obtain an independent account of the patient's problems and background is regarded as important, and with adolescents it is essential. Many doctors in training have commented after a first interview with an adolescent that they really cannot see why the youngster has been referred, only to wonder how they could have been so naive when a parent unfolds a tale of lying, stealing and serious anti-social behaviour. Diagnosis and formulation should not be made until an independent account of this sort has been obtained. In addition, permission for a school report (if appropriate) should be requested. Special investigations such as psychological testing, an electro-encephalogram (E.E.G. or brain wave test) or laboratory investigations may be necessary to round out and clarify the picture.

The formulation should take into account any possible genetic factors, significant early life experience, the physical, intellectual and emotional features contributing to the presenting picture, and also any special areas of difficulty in the developmental process of adolescence. A treatment plan should then be outlined in detail at this stage, although it may have to be modified from time to time as therapy proceeds.

PRINCIPLES OF TREATMENT

The use of the concept involving symptoms, diagnosis, prognosis and treatment is commonly called 'the medical model'. In some circles it has become fashionable to devalue this, but it has long stood the test of time in many branches of medicine, and psychiatry is no exception. Several recent studies have shown that diagnoses made in childhood and adolescence frequently hold constant in adult life. As pointed out in an earlier chapter, the use of classification aids in the understanding of malfunction. In many instances, if the cause of a disturbance can be uncovered, appropriate and specific treatment measures can be instituted. In Part II of this book the medical model has been used to delineate the nature of the psychiatric problems most commonly encountered in dealing with teenagers and, where enough is known, treatment aimed at attacking the cause will always be the first line of approach. The management of specific illness has been discussed to some extent in Part II and will be developed further in this section.

It has been demonstrated that the treatment of dysfunction can be effective *before* the cause is fully understood, and as an example, the use of lime juice in the Merchant Navy cured scurvy long before its relationship to a deficiency of vitamin C was elucidated. In adolescent psychiatry we are in a similar position, trying to effect a cure when the causative agents are only dimly understood. Many problems appear to be multi-factorial. Some adolescents present with difficulties as a result of the process of maturation, but in others the presenting illness itself gives rise to secondary maturational problems. Just as a paediatrician and a child psychiatrist have to take into account the physical and emotional developmental needs of their patients, so a psychiatrist involved with those in the second decade of life must always have an awareness of the physical and emotional needs of normal adolescence.

In some ways, the adolescent psychiatrist may be likened to an orthopaedic surgeon, who specialises in diseases of bones and joints. Interestingly, the word 'orthopaedic' is derived from the Greek, *ortho* meaning straight, and *paed*, child. While the orthopaedic surgeon attempts to ensure that the child is physically straight, the psychiatrist hopes that his patients will be protected from permanent emotional deformity. The analogy may be taken even further. When a limb is damaged, the surgeon has to assess the degree of support required to ensure healing in the best position. This may range from a simple bandage for a sprain, to plaster of paris or a splint for a broken limb to ensure that the ends join up again in good alignment. Similarly, the psychiatrist may have to assess the degree of stress with which a teenager can cope, support being provided in an out-patient setting, or by removal from difficulties through placement in a residential setting, chosen individually for the degree of control and support it can give to a youngster at a particular period of 'emotional fracture' or difficulty.

Essentially, treatment relates to the alteration of an individual's environment. Traditionally it is customary to examine treatment measures under two headings:

a. Modification of the internal environment, including the use of drugs, other methods of physical treatment, or some forms of behaviour therapy and psychotherapy (individual or group).
b. Modification of the external environment, including alteration of parental attitudes, the use of family therapy, change of school or residential placement.

Although this concept helps to clarify thinking about treatment programmes, the distinction is somewhat artificial as the internal world of the teenager impinges on the external world almost inextricably and vice versa. In the succeeding chapters, treatment methods will be looked at in more detail, with stress on the need for flexibility and individual design. Frequently a combination of methods is required.

18 Physical methods of treatment in adolescent psychiatry

USE OF THERAPEUTIC DRUGS

Drugs are pharmacologically-active substances which may be helpful or harmful according to the way in which they are used. The medical practitioner aims at using drugs for the benefit of the patient and so he has to take into account the action of the drugs upon the human organism and the dose required to produce such an action. Often the beneficial or therapeutic dose and the dose producing unwanted effects (side effects) are close to each other. There is usually a recommended range of dosage of drugs for adults and most texts quote the minimum effective and the safe maximum dose. In children, drugs are usually prescribed in relation to body weight. For adolescents, adult dosage is often appropriate but in prepubertal youngsters and, for example, patients with anorexia nervosa, paediatric dosage may be sufficient. Again in general terms, the side effects of drugs in adolescents are similar to those in adults.

On the whole, less medical use is made of drugs in adolescence than at any other age. This is in part because adolescents are usually extremely healthy. The groups of drugs most commonly used in the treatment of adolescents when this is appropriate by psychiatrists are:

241

1. Hypnotics.
2. Anxiolytic drugs (minor tranquillisers).
3. Major tranquillisers.
4. Anti-depressants.
5. Anti-convulsant drugs (*see* Chapter 16).

Hypnotics
Hypnotics are drugs used to induce sleep (from *hypnos*, the Greek word meaning sleep; *see* Table 6). A low dose also reduces anxiety, but the associated drowsiness makes this group of less use than the anxiolytic agents which are available today. The two major groups of hypnotics are:

a. Barbiturates.
b. Non-barbiturates.

The second group comprises chloral hydrate, dichloralphenazone (Welldorm), nitrazepam (Mogadon), Mandrax (which is a combination of methaqualone 25 mg and the anti-histamine diphenhydramine (Benadryl) 25 mg) amongst others.

Barbiturates
These came into clinical use early in the century. Three types of barbiturates are usually recognised:

i. Short-acting.
ii. Long-acting.
iii. Medium-acting.

Short-acting The short-acting barbiturates are used in anaesthesia and include drugs such as thiopentone (Pentothal). This barbiturate is poorly-absorbed when given by mouth and is therefore given intravenously (*i.e.*, by injection into a vein). For psychiatric purposes it is most frequently used for the technique of abreaction. *This is when a psychiatrist wishes to enable a patient to discuss a particularly traumatic life event which is thought to be giving rise to his emotional symptoms.* The patient is given the intravenous injection of Pentothal in a dose sufficient to reduce the level of consciousness and is then encouraged to focus on significant, emotionally-charged material. Abreaction is used rather infrequently with adolescents. For further details of this technique, readers

TABLE 6
Hypnotics in Common Use

Proper name of drug	Trade name	Preparation	Usual dosage
Barbiturates			
Long-acting:			
Phenobarbitone		15 mg 30 mg 60 mg } tablets	30–60 mg t.d.s.*
Medium-acting:			
Amylobarbitone sodium	Sodium Amytal	60 mg 200 mg } tablets	200–400 mg nocte*
Butobarbitone	Soneryl	100 mg 200 mg 300 mg } tablets	100–200 mg nocte
Pentobarbitone sodium	Nembutal	30 mg 50 mg 100 mg } capsules	100–200 mg nocte
Quinalbarbitone sodium	Seconal	50 mg 100 mg } capsules	100–200 mg nocte
		100 mg 200 mg } capsules	100–200 mg nocte
Quinalbarbitone sodium and Amylobarbitone sodium	Tuinal	100 mg 200 mg } capsules	100–200 mg nocte
Short-acting:			
Thiopentone	Pentothal		
Non-barbiturates			
Chloral hydrate	Noctec	500 mg tablets Syrup	500 mg nocte
Dichloralphenazone	Welldorm	650 mg tablets	650–1,300 mg nocte
Triclofos	Tricloryl	500 mg tablets	
Nitrazepam	Mogadon	5 mg tablets	5–10 mg nocte
Methaqualone and diphenhydramine	Mandrax	Methaqualone 250 mg diphenhydramine 25 mg }	1 tablet nocte

* nocte = at night; t.d.s. = three times a day.

are referred to other texts, for example *Introduction to Physical Treatment in Psychiatry* by W. Sargent and E. Slater.

Long-acting Phenobarbitone is the most commonly used long-acting barbiturate but, although it has a sedative effect, it is not used as a hypnotic, in part because of the slowness of its action. It is most frequently used in juveniles for its anti-convulsant properties to control epilepsy. It can have a markedly depressing effect and for this reason is now out of favour as an anxiolytic agent, and even to some extent as an anti-convulsant.

Medium-acting The medium-acting barbiturates are those most commonly used as hypnotics, for example butobarbitone (Soneryl, 100–300 mg) and amylobarbitone sodium, which is usually prescribed as the sodium salt (Sodium Amytal 200 mg). These drugs are quickly absorbed, the hypnotic action beginning in half-an-hour and lasting six to eight hours. Tuinal is a preparation containing equal amounts of the short-acting quinalbarbitone sodium (Seconal) and the medium-acting amylobarbitone sodium, dose 100–200 mg. This combination was chosen as it was thought that the quinalbarbitone would act slightly more quickly than the amylobarbitone, thus sending the patient to sleep, and then the amylobarbitone would theoretically ensure that the patient would not waken during the night.

Barbiturates continually increased in popularity until the last decade, when newer hypnotics became available. Their chief drawbacks are the risks of abuse and overdose, to both of which adolescents are particularly prone. For this reason, the prescription of barbiturates is best avoided in adolescence, but occasionally, in a particularly disturbed patient, Sodium Amytal combined with a major tranquilliser may be helpful in controlling symptoms in the initial stages, especially where a schizophrenic or a manic illness is present.

Intravenous amylobarbitone may also be of value in acute panic reactions. Judging the dose of barbiturates here may be difficult, if an inadequate dose is given, some adolescents may become uninhibited and instead of the desired somnolence, there may be a period of over-talkativeness. (Relatively rare conditions in adolescence such as porphyrinuria, myasthenia gravis or myxoedema are contra-indications to the use of barbiturates.)

Non-barbiturate hypnotics

Chloral hydrate is a safe and reliable hypnotic which has been in use for just over a hundred years. It is prescribed in liquid form as a syrup which makes it particularly useful for teenagers who are suspected of not taking their tablets. Closely related preparations in tablet form are dichloralphenazone (Welldorm) which is a combination of chloral and phenazone (650 mg tablets), and triclofos (Tricloryl) 500 mg. These are again relatively safe hypnotics, although they may be habit-forming, so, like all hypnotics, they should only be used with good reason, and then briefly.

Nitrazepam (Mogadon) is related to the benzodiazepine group which is discussed under the anxiolytic drugs (below). It is a relatively recent hypnotic which acts rapidly and is comparatively safe.

Methaqualone itself has been used as a hypnotic but is more commonly prescribed in combination with the antihistamine Benadryl and marketed as Mandrax. Use of this drug is to be avoided, because of frequent abuse and because of resuscitation problems after an overdose.

Glutethimide (Doriden) is also better avoided because of the occasional occurrence of peripheral neuritis, a potentially dangerous affliction of the nervous system.

Paraldehyde is a well-tried hypnotic which is safe and quick acting and for this reason is may be of value in a psychiatric emergency, but this is the only occasion when its use can be justified. Intramuscular injection is extremely painful and inflammation is likely to result.

Bromide-containing hypnotics are now totally avoided because of their strong tendency to produce toxic effects.

Chlormethiazole (Heminevrin), a drug introduced in the treatment of delirium tremens (a condition rarely seen in adolescence) has now come into use generally as a sedative. Unfortunately, there have been definite reports that it can cause severe habituation and thus lead to abuse, so it should not be used routinely.

Anxiolytic ('anxiety-relieving') drugs

These have also been referred to as minor tranquillisers. In general, however, this latter term is best avoided since, as Dr. Lader has pointed out, their effect is not minor and they have little in common with the major tranquillisers to be described later. Certainly, there is less tendency for anxiolytic drugs to produce such major side-effects as those of the major tranquillisers. They are of especial use when patients have symptoms of anxiety and tension, although

they are not effective hypnotics. There is less likelihood of drug
dependence than with barbiturates and they are less dangerous if
taken in excess (see Table 7).

Meprobamate (Equanil) is a drug which was developed from a
muscle relaxant and it was thought that this property would be
useful in relieving the muscle tension commonly seen in anxiety
states. It was used in the 1950s, but has become less popular with
the introduction of the benzodiazepine drugs, which are more effective and have fewer unwanted side effects. However, the newer drug

TABLE 7
Anxiolytic Drugs in Common Use

Proper name	Trade name	Preparation	Usual dosage
Meprobamate	Equanil Miltown Mepavlon	200–400 mg tablets	400 mg t.d.s.*
Benzodiazepines			
Chlordiaze- poxide	Librium	5 mg, 10 mg, 25 mg tablets 5 mg, 10 mg capsules Injection, 100 mg	10 mg t.d.s.
Diazepam	Valium	2 mg, 5 mg, 10 mg tablets 2 mg, 5 mg capsules Syrup, 2 mg Injection, 5 mg	2 mg–10 mg t.d.s.
Lorazepam	Ativan	1 mg, 2·5 mg tablet	1 mg t.d.s.
Medazepam	Nobrium	5 mg, 10 mg capsules	5 mg t.d.s.
Oxazepam	Serenid D	10 mg, 15 mg tablets 30 mg capsules	10 mg t.d.s.
Clonazepam	Rivotril	0·5 mg, 2 mg tablets Injection, 1 mg	1–2 mg t.d.s.
Beta-adrenergic blocking agents			
Oxprenolol	Trasicor	20 mg, 40 mg, 80 mg tablets	40 mg t.d.s.
Propanalol	Inderal	40 mg, 80 mg tablets	40 mg t.d.s.
Benzoctamine	Tacitin	10 mg tablets	10 mg t.d.s.

* t.d.s. = three times a day.

Tybamate which is chemically related to meprobamate, is more effective and has fewer side-effects.

The benzodiazepines

This group of drugs is now the most commonly used of the anxiolytic agents and came into use in the 1960s. It includes chlordiazepoxide (Librium—Roche), usual dose 10 mg thrice daily, diazepam (Valium—Roche), usual dose 5 mg thrice daily, and oxazepam (Serenid D), usual dose 10–15 mg thrice daily.

Nitrazepam (Mogadon) has already been mentioned under the hypnotics.

Chlordiazepoxide was first noted to have an effect in taming aggressive animals and was introduced clinically in the treatment of chronic schizophrenic patients in whom it was found to alleviate anxiety, althought otherwise it helped them relatively little. It was from this observation that the benzodiazepines have been developed in the treatment of neurotic anxiety. Trials indicate that these drugs are superior to barbiturates in alleviating anxiety; in addition, clonazepam and diazepam are effective anti-convulsants and are consequently used in the treatment of epilepsy. Intravenous clonazepam is now the treatment of choice in status epilepticus (see Chapter 16). Diazepam has also been used profitably in combination with behaviour therapy, particularly in desensitisation in the treatment of phobias (see Chapter 19). On a high dose, patients complain of drowsiness and tiredness, as with barbiturates. A state of excitement may be induced in some patient's if the dosage is inappropriate, and some individuals probably have an idiosyncratic reaction to the drug.

Benzoctamine

Benzoctamine is a new drug belonging to a different group whose action resembles that of the benzodiazepines, but in addition it is likely to have a more marked effect on muscle tension.

Beta-adrenergic blocking agents

Drugs in this group include propranolol and oxyprenalol. As described in the section on anxiety states, symptoms such as palpitations, diarrhoea and excessive sweating are the result of over-activity of the sympathetic nervous system. When beta-adrenergic blocking agents became available (originally for the treatment of high blood pressure), it was considered that they might exert a sedative-like action to control these symptoms. This, in fact, was found to be the case and for some patients the beta-adrenergic blocking agents are a useful adjunct to the management of anxiety symptoms.

Major tranquillisers

These drugs are used particularly in the treatment of psychotic illnesses such as schizophrenia and mania, but in lower dosages may be used as anxiolytic drugs or as an aid to controlling symptoms of aggression. Drugs of this group had been known for many years but were developed in the 1940s, arising from the anti-histamines. There are two main groups of drugs classified as major tranquillisers (*see* Table 8). These are:

a. Phenothiazine derivatives.
b. Butyrophenone derivatives.

The phenothiazine derivatives

These are drugs which depress the activity of the central nervous system, have an action on the peripheral nervous system, and produce extra-pyramidal side-effects. They act as tranquillisers to calm a patient without causing undue drowsiness or, combined with other drugs, may potentiate the effect of those drugs. The phenothiazine nucleus is as illustrated below and, according to the chemical side-chain introduced in the positions marked as R_1 and R_2, the detailed effects of the drug may be altered.

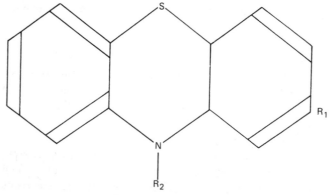

Phenothiazine nucleus

TABLE 8
Major Tranquillisers in Common Use

Proper name	Trade name	Preparation	Usual dosage
Phenothiazines			
Chlorpromazine	Largactil	10, 25, 50, 100 mg tablets Syrup, 25 mg Injection, 10 mg, 25 mg	25–100 mg t.d.s.*
Thioridazine	Melleril	10, 25, 50, 100 mg tablets Syrup 25 mg per 5 ml	25–100 mg t.d.s.
Trifluoperazine	Stelazine	1 mg, 5 mg tablets Capsules 2, 10, 15 mg Injection 1 mg Syrup 1 mg	Up to 15 mg daily. Occasionally greater than this
Fluphenazine	Moditen	1, 2·5, 5 mg tablets Syrup, 0·5 mg	Daily morning dose 2–4 mg
Fluphenazine decaonate	Modecate	25 mg per ml oily injection	25 mg every 2–6 weeks I.M.* Depot injection (see text)
Butyrophenones			
Haloperidol	Serenace	Tablet 1·5 mg, 5 mg 0·5 mg capsule Syrup, 2 mg per ml Injection, 5 mg	0·05 mg/kg body weight for younger patients. 0·5 mg, 1·5 mg t.d.s.

* t.d.s. = three times a day; I.M. = intramuscular injection.

Phenothiazines are classified according to their chemical structure and there are three main groups:

i. Compounds with an *Aliphatic* side chain ending in a dimethylamine group. This group is represented by chlorpromazine (Largactil) which was first introduced into psychiatry by Delay and Denker in 1952. The chemical structure of chlorpromazine appears to make it particularly suitable for overactive, excited or aggressive patients.

ii. Compounds with a side chain ending in piperidine ring, for example, thioridazine (Melleril). These have similar effects to the previous group.

iii. Compounds with a side chain ending in piperazine, for example, trifluoperazine (Stelazine) and perphenazine (Fentazin). Members of this group are thought to have a more activating effect than chlorpromazine and are considered particularly suitable for the more withdrawn schizophrenic patient. These drugs are prescribed in lower dosage than chlorpromazine and thioridazine since they are relatively more potent. Placing a chlorine or fluorine atom in place of a hydrogen atom in the R_1 position increases the stimulating effect of a phenothiazine but is likely to produce a marked increase in extra-pyramidal side-effects (*see* below).

The phenothiazine group of drugs can be given by mouth, intramuscular injection or intravenous injection in divided doses throughout the day. Fairly recently one drug, fluphenazine, has become available as fluphenazine enanthate and fluphenazine decaonate. These preparations are given as a 'depot' intramuscular injection and have a sustained action so that for example, a dose of 25 mg in 1 ml can control a patient's symptoms for 10 to 28 days. This has been of particular use in patients with schizophrenic illnesses who are liable to overlook taking oral medication, or who may avoid taking it because of delusions about the nature of their drugs.

Side-effects of the major tranquillisers can give rise to concern. The most troublesome of these affect the central nervous system, particularly the part known as the extra-pyramidal system. The resulting 'Parkinsonian' symptoms include rigidity, a coarse tremor of the limbs and excessive salivation. Dystonic (abnormal muscular) reactions involve contractions of localised groups of muscles, those particularly affected being in the face, neck and shoulders, but oculogyric spasms (abnormal eye movements) and opisthotonus, in which the patient's back may become acutely arched, can be particularly frightening. Occasionally, a therapist, inexperienced with these drugs, may not recognise such symptoms as side-effects but regard them as abnormal emotional manifestations. Then a further dose of the phenothiazine preparation may be prescribed to 'combat' them, when in fact, the treatment should be an anti-Parkinsonian drug such as biperiden hydrochloride (Akineton) or procyclidine hydrochloride (Kemadrin). These latter drugs are available for intravenous injection when

Parkinsonian symptoms are acute. Akathisia is a term used to describe excessive restlessness, which may be another unwanted effect of phenothiazine drugs. The patient finds it impossible to sit still but the symptom is usually confined to the lower limbs. Once again, this restlessness may be misdiagnosed as agitation and further doses of phenothiazine mistakenly prescribed, so clearly one must always be aware of its possibility.

Although the phenothiazine drugs have a depressant effect on the central nervous system they also lower the convulsive threshold and epileptic attacks may occasionally occur in predisposed persons; therefore, for known epileptics, it may be wise to increase their usual dose of anti-convulsant drugs if they have to receive a phenothiazine in addition.

Other possible side-effects include drowsiness, dryness of the mouth, constipation and weight gain. This last effect has resulted in the drug being introduced into the treatment of anorexia nervosa (*see* Chapter 14). Menstrual irregularity may also occur and many girls who are on phenothiazines have to have their attention drawn to the fact that newly-developed menstrual irregularity is a temporary side-effect of their treatment. Now and again, girls on chlorpromazine may also have false positive response to pregnancy-testing and may require reassurance about this.

In some cases, cardiovascular side-effects are troublesome. These include postural hypotension (when the patient, who has been reclining and then rises suddenly may experience dizziness and weakness and may even faint). These symptoms are said to be more common with those drugs which have to be used in higher dosages, for example chlorpromazine.

The toxic effects of chlorpromazine include skin reactions. These are thought to be more common with chlorpromazine than with other phenothiazines. If a skin rash develops, another phenothiazine may be substituted for the offending drug or, in milder cases, the original may be continued and an anti-histamine added to control the symptoms. Photosensitivity may also be troublesome, particularly with chlorpromazine, in that some patients develop reddening and swelling of the exposed skin when exposed to the sunlight. Agranulocytosis sometimes occurs: this is a failure of the patient to produce a certain type of white cell known as the granulocyte and is a direct, though fortunately rare, complication of chlorpromazine therapy. The patient developing such a condition is likely to present with a sore throat, mouth infection or unexplained high temperature and when any such symptoms occur in a patient on chlorpromazine white blood cell counts should be undertaken as a matter of urgency. Less severe mouth infections are commonly confined to the extremes of life, *i.e.*, to very young children and the elderly, but they have been noted in patients of all ages on phenothiazines, presumably related to the dryness of the mouth which is an irritating side-effect. Jaundice was reported shortly after chlorpromazine was first introduced, but with increasing purity of the preparations used, it is now a rare complication of treatment. It is regarded as an allergic response and is more common with chlorpromazine than with other phenothiazines. For these reasons, chlorpromazine is to be avoided in patients who have a previous history of liver disease. However, having reported all these possible unpleasant complications, it must be said that chlorpromazine and its relatives have been an enormous boon to many ill patients and the incidence of serious side-effects has been very small indeed.

The butyrophenone derivatives

This group of drugs includes haloperiodol (Serenace), trifluperidol and the more recently introduced benperidol. In psychiatric treatment, the effects of these drugs are similar to those of the phenothiazines. They may be prescribed alone or in combination with phenothiazines in the treatment of mania and schizophrenia. In adolescent psychiatry they are also used in the treatment of multiple tics (*see* Chapter 9) and in an attempt to control overactive behaviour. The side-effects of haloperidol and related drugs are similar to those of the phenothiazines but extra-pyramidal effects are common even with small doses so that it is advisable to combine haloperidol with an anti-Parkinsonian, drug from the outset, as these side-effects are particularly distressing. Although haloperidol is still the most commonly used of the butyrophenone derivatives, the very potent trifluperidol is also used. The position of benperidol in clinical practice has yet to be fully evaluated, as it has only recently become available. To date, it has mainly been used in the treatment of uncontrolled anti-social behaviour and sexual disorders and not in the treatment of psychotic illness. It seems to have a fairly specific effect in reducing sexual libido and this may be of value in treating the aggressively disturbed male adolescent who shows sadistic sexual tendencies.

The anti-Parkinsonian drugs

A brief note on these medications might be appropriate here. They are primarily used in general medicine to combat symptoms of neurological illness resulting from disease of the extra-pyramidal system. In psychiatry they have been introduced to control the extrapyramidal side-effects of the phenothiazine and the butyrophenone groups of drugs. The commonly used anti-Parkinsonian drugs are:

Benztropine mesylate (Cogentin)
Benzhexol (Artane)
Biperiden hydrochloride (Akineton)
Procyclidine hydrochloride (Kemadrin)

Psychotic reactions to benzhexol have been occasionally recorded, particularly if a large dose has been prescribed. It was considered that this was more likely to occur in the older patient, but it has also been recognised in psychiatric patients, including adolescents, for whom benzhexol has been prescribed to combat the side-effects of major tranquillisers (*see* Table 9).

The anti-depressant drugs

In the 1950s, reserpine and its derivatives were introduced into clinical practice for the treatment of high blood pressure. It was noted that patients on these drugs sometimes developed markedly depressed moods. It was also observed that reserpine gave rise to a reduction in the concentration of two monoamines in the brain, 5-hydroxytryptamine (5-HT) and noradrenaline. About the same time, doctors were treating patients suffering from tuberculosis with a drug called isoniazid. It was found that one of the side-effects of this drug was an unusual degree of cheerfulness or even euphoria. Further work showed that this and other closely-related drugs did indeed have a beneficial effect on a depressed mood and they have been shown to have the opposite effect to reserpine on the brain, in

TABLE 9
Anti-Parkinsonian Drugs in Common Use

Proper name	Trade name	Preparation	Usual dosage
Benztropine mesylate	Cogentin	2 mg tablets 2 mg Injection	2 mg t.d.s.*
Benhexol	Artane Pipanol	2, 5 mg tablets	2 mg t.d.s.
Procyclidine hydrochloride	Kemadrin	5 mg tablets Injection, 10 mg	2·5–5 mg t.d.s.
Orphenadrine hydrochloride	Disipal	50 mg tablets	50 mg t.d.s.
Biperiden hydrochloride	Akineton	2 mg tablets Injection, 5 mg	2 mg t.d.s.

* t.d.s. = three times a day.

that they produce an increase in the two monoamines already mentioned, 5-HT and noradrenaline. Iproniazid, a close relative of isoniazid, has been shown to act on an enzyme known as monoamine oxidase, which is involved in the metabolism of 5-hydroxytryptamine and noradrenaline, by inactivating it. This group of drugs is therefore known as the monoamine oxidase inhibitors.

With the discovery of chlorpromazine in the early 1950s, doctors searching for further phenothiazine derivatives developed a drug called imipramine. This drug was found to be ineffective in the treatment of schizophrenia, but was shown to act as an antidepressant. Its chemical structure involves three cyclic rings and so imipramine and its derivatives are known as the tricyclic antidepressants. They also act by increasing the available monoamines but in a different way from monoamine oxidase inhibitors. (Readers who are interested in further information on this aspect of neurochemistry should see the references at the end of this chapter.)

Essentially, therefore, two groups of anti-depressant drugs are available:

a. The tricyclic anti-depressants.
b. The monoamine oxidase inhibitors.

In addition, the use of lithium and tryptophan will be discussed (*see* Table 10).

The tricyclic anti-depressants

This group of drugs has been shown to be effective in the treatment of severe depression although it is not as effective as electroconvulsive therapy (E.C.T.) or as rapid in its action, so that E.C.T. still remains the treatment of choice in the actively-suicidal depressed patient (*see* below). It is thought that tricyclics do not attack the root cause of depression, but do correct its disordered biochemistry, so that treatment must be continued until a natural remission occurs. Presumably, related to biochemical changes, it may be up to two weeks before the anti-depressant effect of these drugs becomes apparent and it is important that the patient is informed of this. With adequate dosage, a markedly beneficial effect can usually be obtained after four weeks, but treatment will almost certainly be required for longer than this.

It is on occasion difficult to recognise when remission of the underlying depressive illness has occurred when treatment may be terminated. Sometimes, patients become more aware of discomfort from side-effects when they have improved and no longer need anti-depressant medication. When improvement had been sustained for some weeks, the anti-depressant may be cautiously reduced in dose over the next several weeks. If there is any recurrence of symptoms, dosage at the original level should be reinstituted. Occasionally, it is necessary to continue anti-depressant medication for many months and even for a year. Obviously, it is undesirable for teenagers to be on long-term medication but, for some, this is the only way in which they can cope with life in the community and it is clear that prolonged anti-depressant treatment as an out-patient is better than being an in-patient. Available preparations of the tricyclic anti-depressants are listed in Table 10. It would appear that amytriptyline and trimipramine have a more sedative effect than imipramine and protriptyline, which are said to be more stimulating.

Side effects These include dryness of the mouth, palpitations, visual difficulties related to delay in focussing, fainting, dizziness postural hypotension, vomiting, constipation, urinary retention, sweating and aggravation of pre-existing glaucoma (a potentially dangerous eye-disease).

TABLE 10
Anti-depressants in Common Use

Proper name	Trade name	Preparation	Usual dosage
Tricyclic anti-depressants			
Imipramine	Tofranil	10 mg, 25 mg tablets 25 mg capsules Syrup 25 mg Injection, 25 mg	25–50 mg t.d.s.
Desipramine	Pertofran	25 mg tablets	25–50 mg t.d.s.
Amitriptyline	Laroxyl Saroten Tryptizol Lentizol (long-acting)	10 mg, 25 mg, 50 mg tablets, syrup 10 mg Injection 10 mg Sustained release capsule 25 mg, 50 mg	25–50 mg t.d.s. 50–150 mg t.d.s. 25–100 mg nocte
Nortriptyline	Aventyl Allegron	10 mg, 25 mg tablets Syrup 10 mg	25 mg t.d.s.
Trimipramine	Surmontil	10 mg, 25 mg tablets 50 mg capsule	50–100 mg nocte
Clomipramine	Anafranil	10 mg, 25 mg capsules Syrup 25 mg Injection 25 mg	10–25 mg t.d.s.
Doxepin	Sinequan	10 mg, 25 mg, 50 mg capsules	10–100 mg t.d.s.
Dothiepin	Prothiaden	25 mg capsules	25–50 mg t.d.s.
Protriptyline	Concordin	5 mg, 10 mg tablets	5–20 mg t.d.s.
Monoamine oxidase inhibitors			
Iproniazid	Marsilid	25 mg, 50 mg tablets	50 mg daily
Phenelzine	Nardil	15 mg tablets	15 mg t.d.s.
Isocarboxazid	Marplan	10 mg tablets	10 mg t.d.s.
Tranylcypromine	Parnate	10 mg tablets	10–20 mg t.d.s.
Nialamide	Niamid	25 mg tablets	25–50 mg t.d.s.
Lithium	Camcolit Phasel (sustained release tablet) Priadel (sustained release tablet)	250 mg, 300 mg tablets 400 mg	Based on results of blood level
Tryptrophan	Optimax	500 mg tablets	As prescribed

* t.d.s. = three times daily.

Hypersensitivity to tricyclic anti-depressants may result in skin reactions and blood abnormalities such as agranulocytosis, but fortunately this is rare. Jaundice may occur very occasionally.

Side-effects mediated through the central nervous system include a fine tremor, particularly affecting the upper limbs, or patients may complain of pins and needles or unsteadiness on their feet. The convulsive threshold is altered so that there is an increased predisposition to epilepsy and it may be necessary to increase the dose of anti-convulsants for epileptic patients. Tricyclic anti-depressants are sometimes valuable in the treatment of nocturnal enuresis and it is particularly important in children who suffer from a combination of noctural enuresis and epilepsy, that the tendency for these drugs to lower the convulsive threshold is remembered. Adequate anti-convulsants have to be prescribed to cover the 'small' hours, as it is particularly distressing for parents to be wakened during the night to find a child having a convulsion who has not previously had nocturnal epilepsy. Toxic confusional states have very infrequently been noted when patients are receiving tricyclic anti-depressants. However, once again, it is worth stressing how rare it is to see such serious side-effects.

The monoamineoxidase inhibitors

Once a decision has been made to treat a depressive illness with anti-depressant drugs, most physicians commence with a member of the tricyclic group in view of their relative safety. However, if symptoms fail to respond to a tricyclic anti-depressant they may respond instead to a member of the monoamineoxidase inhibiting group of drugs. Unfortunately, this group of drugs is not without risk, and dietary restriction must be practised to avoid uncomfortable and, occasionally, fatal side-effects. Dietary restrictions are irritating to adults and whereas children's diets can be watched fairly closely, they may be difficult for adolescents whose tolerance of frustration is already lowered by the depressive symptoms and where further irritation relating to food intake may be more than they can bear. Sometimes the youngster himself may exercise care with his diet, but it is not unknown for a jocular friend to play a practical joke and secrete a forbidden food substance in sandwiches, therefore, the decision to use a member of this group of drugs in adolescents requires considerable thought and they should only be prescribed when other measures have failed. For preparations *see* Table 10.

Side effects These include dryness of the mouth, postural hypotension, constipation and dizziness. Water retention is common and can give rise to troublesome swelling of the ankles which is not relieved by diuretics. Skin rashes have sometimes been recorded. A state similar to elation, in which patients have become over-talkative, irritable and disinhibited in behaviour, has been described so that simultaneous treatment with chlorpromazine may be required. Schizophrenic symptoms (which may have gone un-recognised till then) may also be aggravated by monoamineoxidase inhibitors. As with tricyclic anti-depressants, toxic confusional states have been recorded but blood abnormalities are rare.

However, the most serious problem with the monoamineoxidase inhibitors is the interaction with certain food stuffs and with other drugs, resulting in a 'hypertensive crisis'. This is a sudden, acute rise in blood pressure which may give rise to nothing worse than a severe headache but sometimes the outcome may be brain haemorrhage and even death. It is known that these crises are provoked by foods containing the amino-acid tyramine. The foodstuffs most likely to give rise to a hypertensive crisis are:

1. Cheese.
2. Yeast extract (*e.g.,* Marmite and Bovril).
3. Pickled herrings.
4. Alcohol—although one hopes this should not present a problem to younger adolescents!

These foodstuffs should be prohibited absolutely. Hypertensive crises have been reported after eating whole broad beans, but as the pods are not commonly eaten in this country it is not usual to prohibit the eating of broad beans. Coffee and bananas have also been incriminated, but to a much lesser extent.

Drugs which may interact with the monoamineoxidase inhibitors are:

1. The tricyclic anti-depressants.
2. Amphetamine-like substances.
3. Analgesics such as pethidine and morphine or certain local anaesthetics such as cocaine and procaine.

Some of the monoamine oxidase inhibitors may also potentiate the action of drugs like barbiturates, alcohol, phenothiazines and insulin. It is therefore important that if a patient is being treated with a monoamineoxidase inhibitor he should carry a card stating this fact, so that if he is involved in accident or taken to hospital in an emergency the staff treating him will be aware of the situation and the use of incompatible drugs avoided.

Lithium
The lithium ion first came into use for the treatment of mania in 1949, but on account of major toxic effects fell into disfavour. Since the 1960s, it has been re-introduced, but although occasionally used to gain control of the symptoms in intractable mania, it is more commonly used in the *prevention* of recurring manic and depressive episodes. As it is rare to prescribe lithium unless a patient is having recurring attacks of mood-disturbance at frequent intervals, it is only in exceptional circumstances that the drug is used in adolescents. When it is employed, it is usually prescribed as lithium carbonate, tablets being available in 250 and 300 mg strengths. The dose is controlled by estimating blood levels. A long-acting preparation of lithium carbonate (Priadel) is also available as a 'sustained release' capsule, the dose again being adjusted according to blood levels. Before commencing the patient on lithium, it is essential to ensure that the patient's kidney function is adequate, otherwise dangerous blood levels can build up rapidly.

The actual management of lithium treatment is similar to that for the anti-coagulant group of drugs used in medical practice. It is safest for the younger age group to have daily estimates of lithium until therapeutic levels have been maintained for some days, then blood tests may be taken at decreasing intervals but must always be checked on an out-patient basis every four to six weeks for as long as the patient is maintained on the drug (*see* also page 80).
Side effects These should be looked for and recognised early. There are two groups:

1. Gastrointestinal effects: anorexia, diarrhoea and vomiting.
2. Effects on the central nervous system: drowsiness, increasing giddiness, unsteadiness, a coarse tremor of the extremities and lower jaw, buzzing in the ears, blurred vision, muscular

twitchings proceeding to coma and death. Terminally epileptic attacks may occur. (Such severe symptoms will only occur with severe and uncontrolled overdosage.)

Tryptophan
This preparation was noted in the early 1960s to bring about an increase in brain amines comparable with the action of monoamineoxidase inhibitors and tricyclic anti-depressants, although it has its action at a different stage in the biochemical process. Some workers have found that it has a beneficial effect on patients with a depressive illness but its role in the treatment of depression is not firmly established.

OTHER PHYSICAL METHODS OF TREATMENT

Electro-convulsive therapy
Clinical observations earlier this century suggested (wrongly as it turned out) that epilepsy and schizophrenia were infrequently seen in the same patient. Perhaps rather naively, it was considered that if a schizophrenic could have some form of convulsion, this might be beneficial to his illness. Resulting from these observations, schizophrenia was treated with convulsions which were induced by the injection of certain drugs such as oil of camphor and cardiazol. In 1938, Cerletti and Bini developed a treatment method by which convulsions were produced by the passage of an electric current between electrodes placed on the scalp. This is now known as electro-convulsive therapy (E.C.T.) and today is almost exclusively the method of producing therapeutic seizures. When first introduced, the treatment was given to the patient without any form of anaesthetic, but nowadays the convulsion is modified by a muscle-relaxant administered when the patient has been anaesthetised, preferably by a trained anaesthetist.

Indications for E.C.T.
1. Severe depressive illness which has failed to respond to anti-depressant drugs.
2. Schizophrenic illnesses where catatonic features are apparent and where the schizophrenia is acute and is characterised by features of mood disturbance (affective symptoms).

It is the author's impression that the response to E.C.T. is rather less dramatic in teenagers than in adult patients and it is important that young patients are not allowed to become distressed when their response is less rapid than that achieved by adult patients, having the same treatment.

Administration of E.C.T.

The patient is prepared as for any anaesthetic. He should have been fasting over night, as the treatment is usually administered in the morning. Jewellery, dentures and hairclips should be removed and clothing should be loose, particularly around the neck and the waist. An injection of atropine sulphate (0·6–1 mg) is injected intramuscularly half-an-hour before (or intravenously just before) the anaesthetic is commenced. This is a standard pre-medication to ensure that secretions, especially saliva, are temporarily dried up.

The anaesthetic is usually a barbiturate such as thiopentone which is given intravenously, followed by a muscle relaxant such as succinylcholine, but the actual details of the anaesthetic rest with the anesthetist. When the patient is unconscious, a mouth gag is fitted to give a clear airway and to prevent the tongue from being bitten. The E.C.T. is administered through two electrodes which are placed one on each side of the head (bilateral E.C.T.—*see* also unilateral E.C.T. below). The electrodes are circular metal discs covered with lint which has been moistened with saline. They are attached to a head-piece which in turn is linked to the machine which delivers the current. This machine is designed to deliver an alternating current and the voltage and the time for which the current is passed can be regulated. The current which passes through the electrodes is just sufficient to produce a convulsion, but this is modified by the muscle-relaxant so that only slight twitching of the body musculature is seen. When the patient is seen to be jerking a little, the nurses gently hold down his pelvis and shoulders to reduce the risk of any injury occurring.

E.C.T. is usually given twice a week, the length of the course depending on the individual patient's response to treatment. No improvements may be noted until the patient has had about three treatments and it is important to discuss this with him beforehand, as otherwise he may be upset by the lack of noticeable improvement following the first treatment. Usually six to eight treatments are required and it is rare to give more than twelve in a single course.

Despite its apparently severe nature, E.C.T. is a particularly safe form of treatment, but should any serious complication arise it is most likely to occur during the immediate recovery period, so careful observation is required then. As the patient recovers he is likely to be confused and may have some degree of temporary memory disturbance. To reduce this memory loss unilateral E.C.T. has been introduced. In this method both electrodes are applied to the same side of the head, the scalp over the non-dominant cerebral hemisphere being selected. Most of the current avoids the dominant hemisphere in which memory mechanisms are particularly important.

Complications of E.C.T. are rare; the commonest are:

1. Anaesthetic complications.
2. Fractures and dislocations.
3. Dislodging of loose teeth and small cuts to lips.
4. Burns of the scalp if the electrodes and skin are not properly prepared.

These complications are more likely to occur in the elderly than in healthy teenagers and, in any case, relatively few adolescents receive E.C.T.

Psycho-surgery (pre-frontal leucotomy or lobotomy)

Surgical treatment of mental disorder dates back to the mid-1930s, when a Portuguese, Egas Moniz, reported on operations carried out on the pre-frontal lobes of the brains of twenty patients suffering from intractable schizophrenia. From the medical literature, it would appear that the outcry which arose over this form of surgery was similar to that relating to transplant surgery at the present time. There were active protagonists and antagonists, but when pre-frontal leucotomy was introduced it was undoubtedly used by some doctors with too much enthusiasm. A wrongly-inspired or badly-performed operation may produce no benefit at all, or may precipitate such severe personality changes that the patient is worse off than previously. There were many tragic results, including a not inconsiderable number of young people, who were rendered virtually vegetables, or whose behaviour, as a result of the operation, became uninhibited or uncontrollable. Nowadays, the operation is a precision one, used on a small number of highly selected patients, who have been thoroughly assessed.

Psycho-surgery is rarely indicated in adolescence and perhaps the only reason to submit a patient to leucotomy in this age period would be a severe obsessional illness, which had not responded to treatment and which was accompanied by intolerable tension. Dr. Warren, in his follow-up study of adolescents, noted that one of his patients suffering from an obsessional neurosis had had a leucotomy. Dr. Marks and his colleagues reviewed the histories of twenty-four patients, who had had a modified leucotomy on account of anxiety with severe obsessions, and compared them with a group of thirteen matched controls some five years after treatment. They noted that the leucotomy patients had done better than the controls with regard to both obsessions and anxiety, some degree of improvement occurring within three months of the operation. In these circumstances, leucotomy is sometimes a valuable and, occasionally, a life-saving operation procedure, since the adolescent, with a severe and unremitting tension state, may eventually be driven to suicide.

REFERENCES AND FURTHER READING

Anderson, E. W. and Trethowan, W. H. *Psychiatry* (Chapter 22). Ballière Tindall, London, 1973. 3rd Edtn.

Crammer, J. L. (Ed.) *Practical Treatment in Psychiatry*. Blackwell Scientific Publications 1968.

Dally, P. *Chemotherapy of Psychiatric Disorder*. Logos Press, 1967.

Editorial. 'Psycho-Surgery.' Lancet, 1972, *2*, 69.

Levy, R. 'Electro-convulsive Therapy.' Brit. J. Hosp. Med. 1969, *2*, 625.

Silverstone, T. and Turner, P. *Drug Treatment in Psychiatry*. Routledge and Kegan Paul, 1974.

Sargent, W. and Slater, E. *An Introduction to Physical Methods of Treatment in Psychiatry*. 1972. 5th Edtn.

Tan, E., Marks, I. M. and Marset, P. 'Bi-medial Leucotomy in Obsessive Compulsive Neurosis: A Controlled Serial Enquiry.' Brit. J. Psych., 1971, *118*, 155.

Warren, W. 'Study of Psychiatric Adolescent In-Patient and the Outcome Six or More Years Later—II. Follow-Up Study.' Journal Child Psychol & Psychiat., 1965, *6*, 141.

19 Psychological methods of treatment in adolescent psychiatry

Physical methods of treatment have come to the fore in the management of schizophrenia and affective illnesses in the last forty years, but for more than a hundred years increasing attempts have been made to tackle psychologically the problems giving rise to emotional distress.

HISTORICAL INTRODUCTION

In Paris towards the end of the last century, the neurologist Charcot developed a keen interest in patients with hysteria and began to use hypnosis in the treatment of many hysterical patients. Pierre Janet, another famous neurologist of this time, was also interested in the use of hypnosis. Sigmund Freud came under the influence of these two authorities when he visited Paris and, on his return to Vienna, he became increasingly involved with patients with psychiatric illness. Over the years he developed his own psychoanalytic theory of the development of personality, which has been referred to in earlier chapters. This theory has become classical and, even although, with the passage of time, psychoanalytic theory has been considerably modified by Freud's successors, it cannot be denied that he gave tremendous impetus to the treatment of emotional disorders.

Initially, those using hypnosis had tended to concentrate on the treatment of the presenting symptom of the patient, but Freud considered that behaviour was determined by frustration of unconscious instinctual drives and that the patient ought to be helped by attacking the cause of the symptom rather than the symptom itself. He developed his system of treatment (which is sometimes derogatorily dubbed 'the talking treatment') which we know as psychoanalysis. In psychoanalysis, the patient may see his therapist for as much as an hour a day, five or six days per week, over several years and during these interviews he is encouraged to talk freely about everything that comes into his mind, making no attempt to select or suppress his thoughts. This technique is known as 'free association'. Exploration of this and of the material produced from the patient's dreams and interpretation of these are fundamental aspects of psychoanalysis. The relationship between the patient and his therapist, which is known as the 'transference', is regarded as being of particular importance and the positive and negative feeling of the patient for his therapist, and conversely of the therapist for the patient are also examined. Through the therapeutic relationship which he has with his analyst and the interpretation of material produced in therapy, the emotionally-disturbed patient is helped to understand his problems concerning relationships with other people and the particular defence mechanisms which he over-employs. Through the acquisition of insight (which is defined as the emotional understanding of the facts contributing to his difficulties) he may be able to develop a less maladaptive pattern of behaviour than previously.

There are obvious reality limitations to psychoanalysis, in view of the fact that it is expensive and time-consuming, but it has also been found that only selected patients can benefit and, in particular, those of limited intelligence are not regarded as suitable for this therapy. Such drawbacks led many of Freud's followers to look for alternative forms of psychotherapy which would be less expensive in terms of time and resources. Alternative approaches have been developed by a series of workers sometimes known as the neo-Freudians, for example, Erich Fromm, Karen Horney, and Harry Stack Sullivan. They have differed from Freud in some of their theoretical concepts and in general place less emphasis on the importance of the sexual instinct than Freud did. In the various types of analytically-orientated psychotherapy which they have developed, the therapist intervenes more actively in the interview situation, although still making use of free-association and dream-interpretation. He also attempts to direct the content of the therapy session by helping the patients to focus on emotionally-charged areas which are thought to have been of importance in the development of the symptoms. The late Jacob Finesinger developed a particularly useful method of 'goal-directed' insight-therapy and a further development was that of Carl Roger's 'client-centred' psychotherapy, where the emphasis is mostly on the present life-situation rather than past experience. In most of these therapies free association is not employed and the transference is not interpreted, but rather the therapist acts as a 'mirror' for the patient, helping him to identify his own areas of strength and weakness.

As always, there are swings of the pendulum and since the 1950s there has been a swing away from heavy reliance on formal psychotherapy. Behavioural therapy, which is based largely on learning theory, will be considered in more detail below. It is to a considerable extent the application of knowledge gained from experimental psychology in the field of psychiatric disorder. Although it is now well established, behaviour therapy is still regarded as controversial by some people and is, unjustifiably, seen as antagonistic to to other forms of psychotherapy. With greater knowledge about the indications for its use, selection of patients who will undoubtedly benefit from this form of treatment is being more closely defined.

Psychological methods of treatment, though still inefficient in many ways, are gradually becoming more specific in their application and more amenable to accurate assessment of their results.

From the foregoing it will be seen that there are two main forms of psychological treatment:

1. Psychotherapy based on psychodynamic (psychoanalytic) theory.
2. Behaviour therapy based on learning theory.

Each of these forms of treatment includes a variety of methods.

PSYCHOTHERAPY

a. Individual psychotherapy.
b. Group psychotherapy.
c. Conjoint family therapy.

Individual psychotherapy

As experience grew, psychoanalysts became aware that there would have to be some modification in their treatment methods for the younger age groups. Anna Freud (Sigmund Freud's daughter) and Melanie Klein were two of those who recognised this problem and each developed her own method of child analysis. Their techniques had some of the limitations of adult psychoanalysis, being particularly expensive in terms of time and money. Moreover, the majority of psychoanalysts have found the adolescent age group a particularly difficult one to treat and it has been suggested that adolescents who require psychoanalysis should have it deferred until early adult life. However, many psychiatrists working with teenagers do undertake individual psychotherapy, usually based on techniques similar to those described by Rogers in his *Client-Centred Therapy*. A resumé of this is given by Irving Weiner in the chapter on psychotherapy in his text *Psychological Disturbance in Adolescence* and Donald Holmes gave a more detailed account of treatment in his work *The Adolescent in Psychotherapy*. It is only possible to refer briefly here to psychotherapeutic work with the adolescent. In general, this involves dealing with the 'here and now', helping the adolescent to evaluate his strengths and weaknesses, finding ways to bolster up his assets and minimise his defects, helping him to find the opportunities to test out his skills in the environment and so add to his positive experience of life. Whereas, with an adult patient, the therapist can make use of a store of life-experience, it may be necessary for the adolescent to add to his experience in the course of treatment. Often, it is a nice judgment deciding which stage of maturity the teenager has reached and what degree of reality-testing he can withstand. Then, too, adult patients may put themselves to some inconvenience to see the doctor or the social worker and have some understanding of the help that the professional worker is attempting to give, but the professional has to 'sell' himself to the adolescent. He has to work to engage the young person and establish motivation and here the first interview is all-important. It is necessary to form a therapeutic relationship which is challenging, but not critical. The worker has the additional dilemma of deciding whether the teenager should be allowed to see himself in the sick role, or whether this may undermine useful defences he has already built up.

The therapist must show an acceptance of the teenager in all aspects of his personality and communicate a feeling of respect. One needs to be a mature person to cope with being laughed at and this is a particulary traumatic area for a sensitive teenager. Should the therapist feel that a little humour might lighten the situation, he must be able to convey to the teenager that he is laughing with him and not at him. At this stage, assessment must be made of the teenager's level of sophistication, firstly in the social sense, and also of his intellectual and emotional maturity.

Many teenagers wear metaphorical 'suits of armour' and they may be conveniently divided into two groups:

i. Those who are shy, sensitive and lacking in self-confidence, but who basically have sound personalities which can achieve reasonable development. For these teenagers the task is to build up self-esteem so that their excessive defences can gradually be shed as their anxiety lessens.
ii. Secondly, there is the rather inadequate youngster who is emotionally vulnerable and unlikely ever to manifest great personality strength. Here, the aim must be to help strengthen his natural defences so that his inadequacies are not exposed to public gaze, as it may have to be accepted that the inadequacies are largely irreparable.

Bearing the assessment in mind, the psychotherapeutic goal should then be examined. The depth of treatment, that is, the extent to which the patient's defences should be probed, is decided upon. Any attempt to interfere with the adolescent's defence mechanisms is usually too threatening to him and most treatments are best aimed at helping the adolescent to look at his current life-situation and to ascertain to what extent his present behavioural patterns are either adaptive or mal-adaptive. In work with adults, the production of material and the amount of non-verbal communication is largely under the control of the patient, but adolescents tend to become anxious if there are, for example, prolonged silences, so that the therapist has to intervene more than he would with older patients.

As psychotherapy proceeds and the therapist's goals for the youngster are achieved, the tailing-off of the supportive relationship must receive adequate consideration and the young person will require to be 'weaned' out of the situation by decreasing the frequency of contact. The timing of this process can often be dictated by the teenager himself, by perhaps saying 'When do you think I should see you again?' or perhaps offering two appointments, one at a much later date than the other, to see which the patient will select. Teenagers need the opportunity to look at their emotional 'nakedness', but it is only after some time, when they feel that they have the respect of the therapist and can, in return, respect him, that they are prepared to look at their problems. For many teenagers, therefore, individual psychotherapy is the treatment of choice. It is certainly so in the initial stages, when adolescents are referred on account of problems relating to psycho-sexual development or doubts concerning body image. However, there are other adolescents whose difficulties appear to be mainly in the field of interpersonal relationships and many of these benefit from:

Group psychotherapy
The impetus for group psychotherapy in the United Kingdom largely developed during the Second World War. Prior to this, there had been an increasing interest in sociological observations of group culture. In the course of the war, group methods of assessment of candidates for commissions in the armed forces were introduced and, later, prisoners of war undergoing repatriation were exposed to a group situation, in an attempt to facilitate their rehabilitation back into the community. Gradually, psychotherapists became involved in group methods and when an interest was taken by psychoanalysts, the formation of psychotherapeutic groups for the benefit of psychiatric patients occurred.

Group therapy is of particular value for patients who have marked difficulties in interpersonal relationships. However, a group composed of nothing but withdrawn, inhibited teenagers can be a very painful experience for all concerned, so it is important to ensure that it contains a mixture of personalities. In addition, it is recognised that group therapy may be of value in providing relief for patients with anxiety and irrational fears. It has been suggested that changes brought about by treatment in a group situation are longer lasting than those produced by other methods.

Group therapy is based on the developments which arise when a small group of patients meets with a trained group conductor over a period of time, the aim being to bring about changes in behaviour and personality. Strictly speaking this is 'small' group psychotherapy, in contrast to 'large' group therapy which will be mentioned later. A group may be 'open' or 'closed', in the sense that patients may join at any stage of the life of the group or else, once the group commences to function, no new members may join. There are two main schools of thought relating to group therapy. Firstly, are those who see it as an extension of psychoanalytic therapy, the psychiatrist being the group conductor and making use of the transference relationship between him and the group members, the interpretations being based on psychoanalytic theory. Secondly, are those who regard group psychotherapy as a distinct treatment method, in which the relationship between the individual group members is at least as important as the relationships between the patient and the conductor. The latter mainly monitors the inter-relationships and intervenes to influence group interaction. In fact, both approaches can be valid in particular circumstances.

In their move towards independence, adolescents tend to reject adult standards and this can create difficulties in individual psychotherapy, where the therapist may be regarded as a parent-figure and the teenager may be resistant to treatment by him. On the other hand, he may be considerably influenced by peer-group pressures and group psychotherapy is therefore used in many teenage institutions, such as community schools and schools for the maladjusted. Therapeutic groups will normally consist of eight to ten patients, with a therapist and possibly a co-therapist. Should the therapist have any anxieties about his ability to control the group, a co-therapist is advisable, as an insecure conductor may inadvertently encourage acting-out behaviour. Teenage patients should be encouraged to regard material produced in the group setting as confidential. There is no real check on this in out-patient practice, but presumably if the outside community does not know who the other group members are, there is little risk in passing on confidences. However, in the institutional setting there is always a danger that a youngster who has confided his fears in the group situation will be deliberately exposed to the feared situation by any bullies in the group. Initially, teenagers tend to remain anxious and it is a common experience that for ten to twelve weeks the material discussed will have a low emotional tone. Then, as the participants get to know each other and there is increasing confidence, they are prepared to discuss emotional problems in more depth. It is important that the conductor should not be made disheartened or impatient by this, as he may in fact delay the 'gelling' process if his impatience becomes apparent, and is understood by the group for what it is.

Groups for parents of teenagers have also been found helpful, encouraging parents to examine various ways of handling developing youngsters and finding that the difficulties are shared by others.

Large-group therapy
In some establishments, where staff and patients had come to know each other closely, it was considered that their inter-personal relationships could be made use of in the treatment situation and the so-called 'therapeutic community' came into being after the Second World War. This extended the concept of individual psychotherapy, where the aim of building up a relationship between patient and therapist is limited to the therapeutic hour. In the therapeutic community, treatment continues throughout the day and encounters between individuals, and episodes of behaviour, can be examined in a group setting. This type of treatment has been found to be particularly useful for those with acting-out behaviour but it can be destructive for the sensitive, inhibited personality. Therefore, when considering patients for units where large-group therapy is used as an adjunct to treatment, patient selection is very important. It is doubtful if it should ever be used as the only form of treatment in the adolescent age group.

Conjoint family therapy
Traditionally, in the child-guidance setting, psychiatrists worked

with the identified patient, that is, the child, while the highly trained psychiatric social worker would usually work with the parent or parents. Often, 'parent' simply meant the mother, as it was not a practical proposition for the father to have regular time out of work. Increasingly, the importance of father in the family became recognised and, following the Second World War, a form of family-group therapy developed. The basis for this type of therapy is the observation that, although the referred individual has been identified as the patient, he may in fact be a member of a sick family, so that only by helping the family to come to terms with its collective neurosis can the individual himself be helped. On these grounds, in a few areas of the country, family-group therapy has now become the only form of psychotherapeutic treatment offered.

From the outset, the family is seen as a group and the assessment of the problems of the individual at a diagnostic interview (as outlined earlier in this text) is omitted. This is an acceptable practice where a family has been referred by a trained professional worker, specifically for family-therapy, but where there has been no preliminary screening by such a trained professional, it seems undesirable that conjoint family therapy should be the *only* type of treatment offered. This is particularly so in the adolescent age-group, as certain teenagers may have problems, for example, in the area of psycho-sexual development, which it would be difficult and, indeed, inappropriate, for them to discuss in the family setting. Similarly, for those teenagers who are tempted to break away from the family, forcing them back into the family situation cannot always be regarded as beneficial. On the other hand, for certain impulsive teenagers who present with the acting-out of their impulses and who may be 'scapegoated' by their families on account of this, joint family sessions may be particularly helpful, the whole family being encouraged to examine the ways in which it functions.

Family therapy is a relatively new treatment and its final place as a therapeutic tool has yet to be established. It very certainly has its uses, but like any other therapy it also has its limitations. At present, there is a danger that it will be 'over-sold' by the enthusiasm of some of its practitioners and it would be a pity if it got a bad name because it was sometimes employed inappropriately.

BEHAVIOUR THERAPY

In the chapter on conduct disorder, stress was laid on examination of the individual's capacity to learn and of the learning environment. Currently, there is increasing interest in the principles which govern human learning and enquiry in particular into the learning of socially acceptable behaviour, or the reasons for failure to learn such a pattern. Behaviour therapy derives from psychological research into principles of learning and from this research a group of therapeutic techniques has been derived. Reported early work which paved the way to modern learning theory relates to the work of Pavlov, Hull and Skinner and from their studies, theories of classical conditioning and instrumental conditioning arise.

Conditioning procedures

'Classical' conditioning was first observed and investigated by Pavlov in the 1920s. It was known that a hungry dog would salivate at the taste or smell of food and this is termed the 'unconditioned' reflex. If a bell is rung before the food is presented, the dog learns to commence salivating at the sound of the bell, the salivation then being regarded as a 'conditioned' reflex. Subsequently, if the bell is sounded and no food is provided, the dog will salivate as soon as he hears the bell, so the bell has become a 'conditioned stimulus' which evokes the conditioned response of salivation. It has been possible to extend the work with dogs to higher species of the animal world and even to humans. Extensive knowledge is now available about the way in which conditioned reflexes may be produced and how they can become more generalised responses. Readers are referred to Meyer and Chesser's text, *Behaviour Therapy in Clinical Psychiatry* for a more detailed discussion.

Even unsophisticated experimenters became aware that classical conditioning was a gross over-simplication of the learning situation. Thorndyke and Skinner introduced instrumental, or 'operant', conditioning, in which the animal's own behaviour and the presentation of the unconditioned stimulus were arranged in experimental conditions in such a way that the response to be conditioned had to occur *before* the unconditioned stimulus was presented. Thus it was instrumental in producing the unconditioned stimulus. This type of conditioning has indeed long been used, albeit intuitively, by parents and teachers and trainers of animals, for example, in training a dog to shake hands and rewarding him with a titbit subsequently. A system of child-rearing in which many parents will reward acceptable behaviour and show disapproval (or actively punish) unacceptable behaviour is common knowledge, but psychologists observe these phenomena under controlled conditions and try to find an optimum situation and method. The psychologist is also in a position to tackle one aspect of mal-adaptive behaviour in isolation, and is not emotionally involved with the patient to the extent that the parent is with his offspring. But here also lies a potential danger, in that there is a great gap between the laboratory situation and the clinical situation. Initially, most work had been carried out on animals and considerable doubt was expressed by psychologists themselves about the revelance of their experience in the human field. However, there is now a large body of knowledge built up about the value of behaviour therapy in clinical psychiatry. Behaviour therapy is most commonly used in the treatment of neurotic disorders, particularly phobias, psychosexual disorders, certain other developmental disorders such as enuresis and tics and it has also been used in an attempt to gain control of some psychotic symptoms. In current use are a number of techniques, as follows:

   i. Desensitisation therapy.
  ii. Positive conditioning.
 iii. Aversion therapy.
 iv. Negative practice.
  v. Flooding (implosion) therapy.
 vi. Operant conditioning.

Desensitisation
Desensitisation is actually one of the oldest methods of psychological treatment. Mary Cover Jones, in 1924, described the treatment of a young child called Peter, who had a fear of rabbits. He was given some food to allay his anxiety and whilst he was eating, a rabbit in a cage was introduced into the room. Gradually, the cage was brought closer to Peter and eventually the rabbit was released from the cage. Peter was able to tolerate its presence whilst he continued to eat, since eating is a response which is not normally

associated with anxiety. Similar principles are used in the treatment of many phobias and, for example, the agoraphobic initially learns to go out with the therapist and then gradually walks increasing distances from the therapist.

Progressing from those observations, the principles on which modern desensitisation is based have now become established. Anxiety-evoking stimuli are reduced by being associated with pleasurable or relaxing experiences. In the case of Peter this was easy. Relaxation has been used extensively, but is now considered redundant. The therapist works out with the patient a hierarchy of anxiety-producing situations, from those producing least distress to those arousing panic. The patient gradually works through this hierarchy.

It soon became apparent that, if the therapist always had to accompany the patient into the feared situation, this would be hopelessly time consuming, and with certain fears (such as fear of thunderstorms), the reality situation would occur infrequently. Therefore, a system of desensitisation *in imagination* was derived and for many patients relaxation and desensitisation in imagination form the main part of treatment. In other instances, desensitisation in imagination is also combined with practice *in vivo*. To give one example, a teenager might present with a fear of the classroom situation. Considerable time will be spent in obtaining a detailed history and building up a 'hierarchy' of increasingly-feared situations. In this situation, for instance, being in the room with one or two friends might be less anxiety-provoking than being there with the total class. The presence of the teacher might increase or reduce anxiety and this would have to be established. The teenager is then taught deep muscular relaxation over several sessions and, following this, is asked to imagine himself in the feared situation, commencing with a fear at the bottom of the anxiety hierarchy. Initially, some adolescents have great difficulty in imagining situations, but with practice they become more able (or more willing) to do this. In teenagers it is probably more common to introduce them to actual feared situations than it is in adults, rather than relying totally on desensitisation in imagination, and the patient is then given a series of graded tasks to master. Sometimes desensitisation is combined with the use of anxiety-relieving drugs as mentioned in the previous chapter.

Desensitisation has been found to be of particular value in simple phobias and of rather less value in the treatment of agoraphobia and obsessional fears. In instances where there are obviously also major problems in inter-personal relationships, it is sometimes advisable to tackle these aspects by psychotherapy and then, if necessary, move on to desensitisation for the treatment of the phobic disorder.

Many teenagers benefit from 'assertive' therapy in association with desensitisation. This usually takes the form of role-playing, in which the teenager is put into a situation where perhaps he has been criticised in ways he regards as being unfair and he is then systematically encouraged to express his point of view appropriately. This can be a very useful adjunct to other treatment in an introverted and demoralised youngster.

Positive conditioning

This method is particularly used in the bell-and-pad treatment of enuresis as described in Chapter 9 which, it has been suggested, is an example of classical conditioning. The reader will recall that in this method of treatment the patient has two wire mattresses beneath the bottom sheet and these are attached by leads to an electric bell, the circuit being completed when the electrolyte-containing fluid—the urine—wets the top sheet. The bell rings, awakening the patient. In classical conditioning terms, it is considered that the bell is the unconditioned stimulus, the bladder distension which provokes the wetting is the conditioned stimulus, and the waking and the bladder-sphincter contraction together form the response. Ideally, it is hoped that the stimulus of the bladder distension alone will become sufficient to produce bladder-sphincter contraction and thus urinary continence will be achieved. Not all workers accept that classical conditioning is the theoretical concept on which this treatment is based, but since there is no general concurrence on its theoretical background it seems reasonable to regard it as a form of classical conditioning.

Involuntary movements such as tics have been treated by positive conditioning although tics are more commonly being treated by negative practice, nowadays (*see* below). Stammering has also been treated by principles of positive conditioning, using an externally imposed rhythm such as that from a metronome and instructing the patients to speak in time with the metronome beat. Patients are provided with a portable electronic metronome type of apparatus which can be worn behind the ear in a way similar to a hearing aid. By learning to use the apparatus they can gain confidence and then they are instructed to switch off the machine but to continue speaking as if it were still functioning. Gradually, the machine is withdrawn and, in successful cases, a markedly improved speech function can continue without mechanical assistance.

Aversion therapy

Aversion therapy is probably the best known form of behaviour therapy and is certainly the most controversial. It is rarely used with teenagers and should only be employed after considerable heart-searching by the therapist. However, occasionally, the teenager may prefer this kind of help to the legal sanctions which may follow should he be unable to change an abnormal pattern of behaviour, for example, paedophilia (interfering with younger children). An early use of aversion therapy was in the treatment of alcoholism when nausea and vomiting were induced by the administration of a drug such as Apomorphine or Emetine and this nausea deliberately associated with the drinking of alcohol. It is hoped that a conditioned anxiety-response will come to replace the undesirable behaviour by associating the unpleasant stimulus (nausea and vomiting) with the undesired symptom, in this case alcoholism. In fact, this treatment was not without physical risk, and went out of use. The treatment was then adapted for the treatment of homosexuals, induced vomiting and photographic slides of nude males being purposely associated. In the early 1960s, pharmacological aversion was replaced by the controlled use of a mild electric shock. This was much less dangerous for the patient and it was easier to control the timing and strength of the shock. This type of treatment has been used for patients with fetishism, transvestism, homosexuality and paedophilia. It seems highly important to the author that the therapist should be certain that he is dealing with a fixed sexual deviation before aversive therapy can be justified in the younger age group. As well as this, it must be made clear that this treatment is not some form of torture. It is certainly unpleasant, but it is unavoidably used where the patient has a strong desire to co-operate in changing an unwanted form of behaviour.

Negative practice
This type of treatment is based on the principle that massed practice of a learned response without reinforcement leads to extinction. Paediatricians, for example, have been using a method of massed practice in the treatment of tics as far back as the 1930s. The child with tics was encouraged to sit in front of a mirror and consciously and repeatedly to carry out their eye blink or facial tic. Similarly, stammerers have been treated by sessions in which they have attempted to imitate or fake their stammer, but in this particular instance the results have not been very encouraging.

Flooding (implosion) therapy
Observations on animals indicated that if the escape from a conditioned, anxiety-produced stimulus could be prevented or delayed the extinction of the response would speed up. Several theoretical explanations for this observation have been put forward. In the late 1960s a method of treatment based on these observations was developed which is known as 'implosion' therapy. (In other words, the patient fears 'explode inwards'.)

As with the desensitisation method already described, a hierarchy of anxiety-provoking situations is drawn up for each individual patient and the patient is encouraged to imagine that he is in the feared situation. However, in contrast to desensitisation, anxiety is allowed to rise to as high a level as possible. The patient is encouraged to imagine successive items from the hierarchy which evoke anxiety, the least first. This anxiety rises to a maximum then, as it begins to fall, he is encouraged to imagine the next item in the hierarchy. The session should end when the patient's overall anxiety has begun to fall.

In some instances, patients are actually introduced to the anxiety-provoking situation and this technique is particularly useful in patients who have compulsive rituals such as hand-washing where treatment consists of persuading them to wash their hands for long periods of time until their anxiety begins to reduce. It has also been used successfully in treating such diverse phobias as those related to thunderstorms, spiders and enclosed spaces.

Operant conditioning

As described at the beginning of this section on behaviour therapy, operant conditioning is based on instrumental conditioning, such as that described by Skinner in the late 1930s. Although originally derived from laboratory experiments with animals, it has been found that Skinner's work can be applied to the modification of human behaviour. Early work was done with patients who were mentally subnormal, or had a psychotic illness. Decisions were taken as to which particular symptoms were to be modified (the 'target' behaviours). Behaviour was studied so that those environmental factors which rewarded the undesirable behaviour could be identified. A treatment regime was then instituted so that these rewards were withdrawn. In addition, when the patient exhibited a hitherto unused *healthy* form of behaviour, an appropriate and immediate reward (positive reinforcement) was given. Since those early days a large body of experience in the use of the techniques of operant conditioning has been built up. The treatment has been used in the management of autistic children, to help them, amongst other things, to develop useful speech, the reward being, for example, a sweet given initially for any verbal utterance. The reward schedule is then altered to encourage verbal utterance in response to speech from an adult and later, further shaping of the patient's verbal responses is undertaken by rewarding only intelligible utterances. The use of 'group techniques' has also spread to behaviour therapy and a treatment programme known as 'token economy' is in use. It has been particularly useful where it has been possible to treat a group of children with similar symptoms, such as sufferers from childhood psychosis, on the same ward. Desirable activities are reinforced by the use of tokens which can be spent according to the stage of development of the children, for example, on sweets, toys, viewing television, cosmetics and so on. Token-economy systems have been found to be of great use in modifying beneficially the behaviour of sub-normal teenagers and sometimes in classrooms situations and in Community schools.

Attempts have been made to help hyperkinetic children by the use of 'time out'. It was observed that in many hyperkinetics the undesirable behaviour was being reinforced by the amount of attention which the parent or teacher was virtually forced to give to these acting-out children. By altering the approach and ignoring the child's temper tantrums, but noting and actually rewarding socially acceptable behaviour, the number of tantrums or destructive episodes could be considerably reduced. This is sometimes achieved most efficiently by removing the child from the main activity situation and in many establishments there is now a 'time out' room, where the disturbed child may go for a few minutes at a time until he is calmed down. Such treatments are spreading to some primary schools where one particular teacher is involved with the class for most of the day. To initiate similar treatment methods in the secondary school situation is less practical, in view of the large number of adults that the child encounters during a typical school day and also because of the greater influence of the peer group. However, in community homes of the former approved-school type, such treatment programmes have been devised although the degree of success met with has yet to be evaluated.

From the foregoing, it will be apparent that psychological methods of treatment are numerous and that the indications and contra-indications for any particular type are still in the process of being examined. In many instances, more than one type of psychological treatment will be of value in a given patient and these may also be combined with physical methods of treatment. Obviously it is a very exciting time for those involved in the treatment of teenagers with emotional problems, but it is also a time for cool appraisal of our therapeutic approaches, so that we may be sure they are truly effective.

REFERENCES AND FURTHER READING

Balsam, R. M. and Balsam, A. *Becoming a Psychotherapist: A Clinical Primer.* Little, Brown & Company, Boston, 1974.
Crown, S. 'Psychotherapy.' Brit. J. Hosp. Med., 1973 *9*, 355.
Gelder, M. G. 'Behaviour Therapy.' Hosp. Medicine, 1967, *1*, 306.
Holmes, D. *The Adolescent in Psychotherapy.* Little, Brown & Company, Boston, 1964.
Kreeger, L. (Ed.). *Large Group Therapy.* Constable, 1975.
Meyer, V. and Chester, E. S. *Behaviour Therapy in Clinical Psychiatry.* Penguin Books, 1970.
Minuchin, S. *Families and Family Therapy.* Tavistock Publications Ltd., 1974.
Rachman, S. 'Introduction of Behaviour Therapy.' Behav. Res. Ther., 1963, 1.3. Vol. 1, page 3.

Raport, R. N. *Community as a Doctor*. Tavistock Publications, 1960.
Rogers, C. *Client-Centred Therapy*. Houghton Miffelin, 1951.
Skynner, A. C. R. 'A Group-Analytic Approach to Conjoint Family Therapy.' Journal Child Psychol. and Psychiat., 1969, *10*, 81.
Skynner, A. C. R. 'Indications for and against Conjoint Family Therapy.' Social Work Today, 1971, *2*, 3.
Walton, H. (Ed.). *Small-Group Psychotherapy*. Penguin Books, 1971.
Weiner, I. *Psychological Disturbance in Adolescents*. John Wiley & Sons Inc., 1970.

20 Social intervention and residential provision in adolescence

THE SOCIAL WORKER

The writer is aware that throughout this text minimal emphasis has been given to the role of social factors contributing to teenage difficulties, and the impact which a good social worker may make: it is time to make amends for this omission.

In an earlier chapter, reference was made to the adverse effects of material, emotional and cultural deprivation on the developing child, and the repercussions which the insecurity associated with these factors causes in adolescence. The local authority Social Services Departments carry the brunt of the teenage distress resulting from these environmental experiences and the demands placed on the residential social workers and the field social workers employed by these departments are enormous, and with increasing legislation the burden is growing. Yet, as we are identifying those factors contributing to insecurity and resulting instability, the opportunities for preventive work are expanding, but the human and material resources are not.

Much is demanded of the social worker in the 1970s. He needs to know of provision which can improve the material fortunes of the client, and encourage his client to make use of this knowledge to better his position, rather than 'taking over'. The social worker must have an acute awareness of the subtleties of the various sub-cultures with which he comes in contact and use his knowledge to reduce the social isolation of some of the families with whom he is working. Added to these, he is required to have sophisticated casework skills. At an earlier period, as in psychiatry, much casework was based on a psychoanalytically-oriented training and, indeed, many social workers had a more intensive training than some of their psychiatrist colleagues. The modern social worker still has an awareness of, and makes use of, psychodynamic factors in his casework but in addition, will have an understanding of methods of behaviour-modification and will then make use of a combination of methods in his social work skills. Ideally, the social workers in the hospital setting will also have specialised knowledge of the need of psychiatric patients and their families and will use this to help parents understand the implications of psychiatric treatment. As if this were not enough, the social worker who is concerned with adolescents and their families has an important educational role. He has to assist parents in their understanding of the developmental tasks of the adolescent, enabling them to increase the teenagers outlets towards independence when indicated, and control their anxiety when offspring first show an interest in 'the opposite sex'. Thus, the social worker has an important role in the total assessment and treatment situation.

Many social workers have become involved as conductors of small groups in psychotherapy, or in family group therapy. Sometimes doctors, psychologists and social workers work together as co-therapists in such situations.

As with other professional workers, the social worker may often be involved in the community and will work directly with the local authority Social Services Department, or be seconded to work in a hospital psychiatric clinic, a community home or a special school, although in the majority of instances, the social workers in special schools or child guidance clinics are employed by the local authority Education Department.

Since this text is concerned with psychiatric aspects of adolescent problems, it would be invidious to do more than outline the complexities of the social worker's task, but this is not to diminish it.

RESIDENTIAL PROVISION

Occasionally, it may be considered that the home environment is too damaging for the developing teenager and that it is unlikely that beneficial modification of the attitudes in the home environment can be made at all, or in a sufficiently short period of time, to be of advantage to a particular patient. In such instances, placement in a residential establishment may be indicated. This poses the problem of where a given child should go. The decision to remove the teenager from home must never be taken lightly but one it is made, a variety of residential establishments have to be considered, including those provided by:

1. The local authority Social Services Department.
2. The local authority Education Department.
3. The National Health Service.
4. The Department of Health and Social Security, including former Home Office provision.

Residential establishments under the supervision of the local authority Department of Social Services

This department supervises the whole range of community homes. These include the former Children's Homes run by the now-defunct local authority Children's Department, which was amalgamated with the local authority Welfare and Mental Health Departments to become the present local authority Department of Social Services. It also includes the Approved Schools which used to be given a certificate of approval by the Home Office (hence their name), although managed in many instances by voluntary bodies.

Children's homes

Originally Children's Homes, successors to the orphanages, were for individuals in need of a substitute home as the result of the absence of parent or guardian, or because of parental neglect, that is, their role was to replace a deficiency and fulfill a social need. As discussed in Chapter 1, as society has become aware of the effects of sensory, material and emotional deprivation, the large impersonal orphanage has been replaced by Family Group Homes and working boys', or girls' Hostels with the emphasis on maintaining the children's links with the community. Unfortunately, however, many children admitted to the care of the local authority have already suffered serious deprivation, so it is not surprising that many of them have major behavioural problems, when they arrive.

Community homes with residential education
Until the 1969 Children and Young Persons Act, boys and girls were committed to Approved Schools by the Juvenile Court if they failed to respond to, or co-operate with, alternative forms of help like probation or other sanction, such as a fine. Under the 1969 Act, 'Fit Person Orders' (by which a child could be given into the care of a person deemed fit to look after him) and 'Approved School Orders' were replaced by 'Care Orders', under which a child is committed to the care of the local authority, which then has the responsibility of finding a suitable placement for him. This may, but need not necessarily, be, a community home of the former Approved School type.

The Approved Schools have been taken over completely by the local authority Departments of Social Services and have been added to their range of community homes. In contrast to Children's Homes, where the range of ages and sexes tends to be mixed and the children attend the neighbourhood school, youth club, etc., the community schools, so far are single-sex and have been divided into junior, intermediate and senior schools according to age, education actually being provided on the premises, hence the term, community home with residential education. Under the former Approved Schools System there was a range of specialisation in that some schools catered for children of limited ability and others for children of superior intelligence, while others still were geared to help the youngster to prepare for the trade which he might like to follow when older. With reorganisation and regionalisation it remains to be seen whether the Approved School in its new role as a Community Home will be able to provide the degree of selection previously seen.

In the Approved School, a teenager was educated, or had occupational training, within the school, although many had links with outside youth clubs and other neighbourhood contacts. The majority of Approved Schools tended to have a fairly structured day and a wide range of recreational activities was available on site. The provision of such facilities was never cheap and it could cost the community as much to keep a teenager at an Approved School as to keep a boy at a Public School. The vast majority of boys who reached an Approved School did so because of anti-social offences, whereas girls tended to be committed because they were beyond parental control or in need of care and protection. The majority of Approved Schools had a visiting psychiatrist, so that out-patient forms of psychiatric treatment could be undertaken where indicated. In many, staff conducted group therapy with the teenagers, or mixed staff and youngster group meetings were held. At the end of 1970, as the 1969 Children and Young Persons Act was being implemented, there were 124 Approved Schools, of which only 37 were managed by local authorities. The majority of schools were for boys and only 34 were for girls; including what were then called classifying schools; there were 7,930 places available for boys and 1,387 for girls.*

**Establishments under the supervision of the
local authority Education Department**
In this country there is a tradition for children of leading families to be educated at boarding school and many parents will deprive themselves financially in order to give their children the opportunity to go to a Public School. Following the introduction of compulsory education, local education authorities became aware that, for one reason or another, some pupils were unable to benefit from the normal classroom situation, for example, children who are blind, deaf, or have a major physical handicap. In densely populated areas, special day schools were made available, but for the needs of those in rural areas boarding places were required. Another group of children were those regarded as delicate: children admitted to hospital with rheumatic fever might have to return home to a damp, overcrowded house, when they could easily succumb to a further streptococcal infection. This might well cause a recurrence of the rheumatic fever, requiring further admission to a hospital, in an attempt to lessen the risk of cardiac damage. Frequent hospital admissions interrupted these patients' schooling and, while those with cardiac damage were advised to work with their brains rather than

* Figures obtained from *Statistics Relating to Approved Schools, Remand Homes and Attendance Centres in England and Wales for the year 1970.* H.M.S.O. Cmmd. 4879 1972.

brawn, they were seriously handicapped in finding suitable employment because of their lack of education. Hospital schools were established in relation to the children's hospitals and to the children's orthopaedic wards where, before effective anti-tuberculous drugs became available, children might spend many months in hospital on account of tuberculous infection of bones and joint. Day and residential schools were also established for the so-called 'delicate children'. Sometimes these became known as Open-Air Schools; in addition to education there was emphasis on a good diet, adequate rest, and many of them were situated in the open countryside. With the introduction of antibiotics the number of delicate children dwindled and many of these schools consequently had vancanies. In some areas, children with mild emotional disturbance were introduced and today many Open-Air Schools have a number of maladjusted children, particularly those with neurotic complaints.

Another type of special school is for the maladjusted; again, these may be day or residential, pupils having been selected on account of educational difficulties in the normal school streams because of recognisable emotional problems, or psychological disturbance necessitating special educational treatment in order to effect their personal, social and educational readjustment. Prior to the raising of the school leaving age, pupils who were deemed maladjusted were specially required to remain at school, until the age of sixteen. Now of course, this is the rule for all children.

Interestingly, many children at schools for the maladjusted had a longer 'sentence' than children sent to Approved Schools, where the maximum length of stay was three years and was usually much less than this. Theoretically, it is possible for a teenager to be deemed maladjusted until he reaches school-leaving age, but the pressure on places at special schools is such that older children understandably tend to be by-passed in favour of 11 and 12-year-olds. A practical difficulty in relation to residential educational establishments arises when parents find it difficult to contain an individual child during their longer school holidays. Many schools for the maladjusted have a visting psychiatrist, so that, as in Community Homes, individual and group psychotherapy can be available.

Children with limited intelligence may require special educational help; this may be provided in a special stream at the neighbourhood school or at a special day or boarding school. Some years ago, it was considered that children with an intelligence quotient of less than fifty were ineducable and the Local Health Authority provided Junior Training Centres for these children. Now, however, the Junior Training Centres have been taken over by the local education authority and are run as schools for those who are severely mentally handicapped.

Provision similar to that of the local education authority may be provided by various voluntary bodies and many local authorities will make financial arrangements for an individual child to be educated in such an establishment if there is a shortage of vacancies in their own schools. However, independent provision also tends to be over-subscribed, particularly for the older school child.

At any one time, approximately 5,000 children in England and Wales will be deemed maladjusted out of a total of about 130,000 handicapped pupils. Their care and treatment is a very considerable charge on a number of important services.

The following categories of handicapped pupils are recognised, namely:

a. Blind.
b. Partially sighted.
c. Deaf
d. Partially hearing.
e. Physically handicapped.
f. Delicate.
g. Maladjusted.
h. Educationally handicapped.
   Severely educationally handicapped.
i. Epileptic.
j. Speech defect.

National health service provision
Out-patient psychiatric treatment for adolescents has been referred to in Chapter 3. Until shortly after the Second World War, adolescents who required in-patient psychiatric treatment in Britain could only be admitted to adult wards.

Following the epidemic of encephalitis lethargica ('sleepy sickness') after the First World War, many brain-damaged children with behavioural disorders required hospital care. As these children became adolescent and moved on to the adult wards they often become a thorn in the flesh of the adult patients, as is the way of teenagers, and this highlighted the problems of mixing the two age-groups. Also, an adult schizophrenic or alcoholic was considered to be an undesirable model for the developing teenager. For these reasons, it was considered in some hospitals in America that adolescents should be nursed in a ward of their own. There are hair-raising accounts in the medical literature of the difficulties which the staff of the pioneer adolescent units encountered. It is recorded that in one unit the nurses had to retreat inside a wire cage to protect themselves from the missiles of their young charges! At that time, the staff–patient ratio on the adolescent ward at this particular hospital was similar to that on an adult ward. When the number of patients was halved, but the number of staff remained unchanged, it was found that the staff could emerge from their cage without incident. It is for this, among several other reasons, that a high staff–patient ratio is required and why adolescent units are relatively expensive to run.

After the Second World War, the first adolescent unit was opened in the United Kingdom. This was at St. Ebba's Hospital in Epsom (this hospital has now become a mental-subnormality hospital and the adolescent unit has been transferred to Long Grove Hospital). Shortly after, another unit was opened at Bethlem Royal and Maudsley Hospital. Gradually, the number of units throughout the country has increased, impetus being given by a Ministry of Health circular recommending that there should be twenty to twenty-five adolescent psychiatric beds per million of the entire population. Interestingly, the adolescent age range was not defined. More recently, adolescent units have had difficulty in opening because of a shortage of trained staff in all the helping disciplines.

Some existing adolescent units cater for children up to the statutory school-leaving age and there are others that function as Young People's Units, admitting patients aged 16 to 21 years. Those catering for the younger age group usually have a hospital school attached.

However, not all disturbed teenagers falling into this age group are suitable for treatment in adolescent units and selected adolescents may in fact do better on an adult ward. This may be the adult ward of a psychiatric unit in a general hospital, or one in a psychiatric hospital. This will be discussed further, subsequently (*see* page 299). Unfortunately, a few teenagers need more secure conditions than are available at an adolescent unit or a psychiatric hospital and placement in one of the maximum security hospitals may have to be arranged for these.

Department of Health and Social Security
Youth treatment centres
Recently, the Department of Health and Social Security introduced the new concept of Youth Treatment Centres. These were for particularly disturbed children in the care of the local authority who were thought to require a long-term, relatively secure, placement. The first of these Youth Centres is at St. Charles, Brentwood, in Essex, and will eventually cater for fifty boys and girls. It is envisaged that a second centre will open in the Midlands later this decade and a centre is also planned for the north of England.

With this range of provision, how does one select the appropriate place for a given individual? For some teenagers the choice will be clear-cut. A girl with anorexia nervosa will be directed to hospital, while the child with obvious educational difficulties may be placed in a special school. In the past, the local authority Children's Department was aware of the need to select long-term placement with great care and children's Reception Centres were set up where a child was temporarily admitted so that his needs could be assessed. Reports were provided by the Warden of the reception centre, a local authority Social Worker, and possibly also a child psychiatrist and/or a psychologist. After a period of observation a meeting of the professional workers concerned (the case conference) was held and the best available placement for the child under consideration was decided on. This might involve fostering, or placement in a particular children's home.

A Juvenile Court's decision to make an Approved School order would often follow a period of assessment at a Juvenile Remand Centre, which was similar to that carried out at the children's reception centre. Once an Approved School order was made, the boy or girl was moved to what was known as a Classifying School as soon as a vacancy arose. There were five of these in England, Aycliffe and Redbank in the north, Kingswood near Bristol which catered for the Midlands, and Redhill in Surrey and Stamford House in London for the south. Following further assessment, a particular Approved School would be selected.

With the implementation of the 1969 Children and Young Persons Act and with the regionalisation of the former Approved Schools system, in many areas the clientele of the former children's reception and remand centres is becoming less distinct and where there is pressure on places a teenager may simply go to an establishment which happens to have the first vacancy. It is usually after a period of observation and assessment that the Magistrate at the Juvenile Court will make a Care Order committing the child to the care of the local authority. Sometimes when a Care Order is made, the decision regarding placement will be obvious, but in many instances further assessment may be required and for this purpose each region of the country is setting up an assessment centre similar to the former Classifying Schools. Following a further period of observation in such a centre the final placement choice is made.

Selection of the appropriate placement at a residential establishment will often depend on the degree of control that the youngster requires. If he has no history of truancy and is able to take some responsibility for his own behaviour, a family group home for school children or a working boys'/girls' hostel for young school leavers may be suitable. For the adolescent whose behaviour is out of control and who has little in the way of self-discipline, a more structured environment with a carefully planned time-table, and with educational or work facilities available on the premises will be indicated, such as was available at the former Approved Schools. One of the advantages of the 1969 Act is that, on a care order, a teenager may start off in a controlled environment and as he matures he may move to a more permissive regime, such as will become available in each region as a range of community homes becomes established. Often in the past, a teenager moved from an organised day, with supervised leisure at an Approved School, back to a disorganised home environment, commonly in an area of high delinquency, and this was a powerful source of relapse.

By and large, the special residential educational provision is not as structured as that in an Approved School and is more suitable for those adolescents who have some degree of internalised control, but whose emotional problems, rather than their home environment, are a major problem. Sometimes, admission to a hospital adolescent unit may be used for assessment in order to decide

whether a given patient would be better helped by the local authority Department of Social Services or by the Local Education
Authority. The hospital adolescent unit provides twenty-four hour
psychiatric, medical and nursing care, and it is a particularly
expensive resource, so it seems important that patients are not admitted lightly.

Among the skills of a professional worker is learning to understand the client's needs and appreciating the range of establishments available in his area, so that he can give the teenager a
fairly detailed description of life to be expected in a particular establishment. He should also have contact with staff members in
such establishments. On the whole, in the local authority assessment centres, a highly professional assessment is carried out, and
usually a detailed treatment plan or formulation of the child's
needs is made. Ideally, from this assessment, the residential place
best suited to the child's needs is chosen but, sadly, as a result of
shortage and relative inexperience of staff working in residential establishments, the ideal may not be available and only too often a
teenager has to take the available, rather than the best, place. This
is particularly distressing to the professional workers involved who
have spent a lot of time and energy in the process of observation
and assessment.

Control

In 1967, a London borough's working party (*see* Chapter 10)
reported on the lack of provision for the seriously disturbed
adolescent; they noted that, in addition to a marked lack of
facilities, there was also a lack of co-ordination of those facilities
which did exist and a lack of communication between those responsible for the provision of resources, thus hindering both assessment
and rational planning for the long-term needs of the disturbed
adolescent. Unfortunately, almost a decade later, the situation has
changed little. The working party further drew attention to the
adolescent's needs for supervision and thought that when considering placement, the degree of control should be taken into consideration. In addition, they stated that consideration should be
given to:

a. The level of psychiatric medical/nursing care and treatment
   required;

b. the level of disturbance and distress of the young person and his consequent need to be removed from the community;

c. his ability to take part in ordinary life at home, school and at work;

d. lastly, the availability of social care, education and training.

One of the key features in this is a closer examination of the degree of control required. The child who, at an earlier stage of life, succeeded in developing a fairly strong conscience and has well-developed internalised emotional control, is unlikely to need much external control in adolescence, but there are certain children whom it is difficult to treat, as they are continually absconding. The promiscuous girl gets deeper into the mire each time she is away and, sadly, it is often a pregnancy that finally provides the control which she has been implicitly demanding for some time. In England and Wales there have been, for a considerable time, special closed units within the Approved School system. Many of the larger Approved Schools also had a 'house' system in operation, so that for example, the shy, inhibited boy could be kept separate from the overweaning bully and the less intelligent boy could be protected to some extent from major problems relating to his lack of ability. At a Youth Treatment Centre it is proposed that there will be one area under conditions of maximum control (twenty places in all), another where a lesser degree of control will be available and approximately twenty places where control will be minimal. For teenagers who are considered to require maximum control, one of the maximum security hospitals, a closed Approved School or the secure section at St. Charles' Youth Treatment Centre are theoretical possibilities. Ordinary community schools, boarding schools for the maladjusted and psychiatric hospitals, where education and work facilities are available on the premises, all provide a moderate degree of control. It is usually considered that establishments with conditions where the need for control is minimal are the ordinary Children's Homes, with out-patient psychiatric help and attendance at day school.

In removing a youngster from home, it is essential that we should not actually do harm. We must therefore ensure that we have something positive to offer him and it is certainly not to the youngster's advantage for an establishment to be opened which is inadequately staffed, with unskilled workers. This is the way to court disaster and it cannot be sufficiently stressed how much the careful selection of staff and residents is of the essence.

Whilst only a small proportion of disturbed teenagers require residential placement, those who do represent a highly-disturbed group. Until we are able to ensure greater stability in the community, we will continue to be presented with many such problems and unless we can help these youngsters to come to terms with their development, they will certainly, in their turn, transmit their problems to their own children.

REFERENCES AND FURTHER READING

Balbernie, R. *Residential Work with Children.* Pub. 1966, Pergamon Press. Revised Edition, Human Context Books. Chaucer Publishing Co. Ltd.

Beedell, C. *Residential Life with Children.* Routledge & Kegan Paul, 1970.

Department of Health and Social Security. *Youth Treatment Centres. A New Form of Provision for Severely Disturbed Children.* H.M.S.O. 1971.

London Boroughs Association. *Interim Report of Working Party on the Provision for seriously disturbed adolescents.* June 1967.

21 The adolescent in-patient

There are now over thirty units in the British National Health Service specialising in the psychiatric treatment of adolescents. Each has its own character, some units treating girls only and others boys, but the majority cater for both sexes. The age-range varies, some concentrating on the 11 to 16-plus age group (that is, the stage of secondary schooling) while others admit young school leavers and those in continuing education from 16-plus to 21 years. Yet others restrict themselves to teenagers, *i.e.*, 13 to 19 years.

The size of these units also varies, ranging from fifteen to thirty-six beds. In the largest units, it is sometimes a deliberate policy not to fill all the beds as, with a group over thirty, it may be difficult to provide the degree of individual care considered desirable. On the other hand, a unit of fifteen beds, unless for a single sex, may result in some youngsters being rather isolated, as they may not fit in on account of age, emotional maturity, or interests, with the dominant group. In such a small unit as this, a number of withdrawn teenagers and one or two schizophrenic patients may make it all but impossible to have a cohesive and therapeutic group.

The majority of adolescent units cater for a population from a wide geographical area and it is therefore essential that they are convenient to public transport. Also, as teenagers gain more confidence, it may be part of a treatment policy to wean them out into

295

the community, so accessibility to public transport means that it is practicable for them to go to the neighbourhood school or to employment. However, in the majority of units, the framework of the treatment programme is similar to that of a boarding school, the majority of patients spending their day in unit-based activities. In contrast to a boarding school, however, but as with other hospital wards, the adolescent units tend to encourage regular visiting, probably several times weekly, so that the teenager can maintain close contact with his family. This feature is sometimes made use of when one is considering boarding school as a long-term goal, so that a sensitive, dependent teenager can be gradually coaxed away from his family. Also in contrast to boarding school, it may be easier for the patients and parents to see the intention behind the action and perhaps to understand that, once they are sufficiently improved, they will be able to return home and to the community. Admission to an adolescent unit may be part of an on-going treatment programme with out-patient psychotherapy, both preceding and following a period of in-patient treatment.

Duration of stay in an adolescent unit varies considerably. Sometimes parents miss their teenage offspring after a few days and decide to remove him from hospital, or else a manipulative teenager may pressurise his parents into removing him. Few units attempt to provide long-term treatment and it would be unusual for a patient to stay longer than a year. Probably the most common range of treatment period is from three to six months, the stay sometimes being more prolonged because a placement in a special day or boarding school is unavailable on account of long waiting lists, or perhaps because a long summer holiday intervenes. In other instances, it may be unrealistic to expect a patient to return to school for one term before he reaches statutory school-leaving age and so some units agree to a brief prolongation of stay in order to overcome this practical problem.

ADMISSION

In many adolescent units, it is considered desirable for the prospective patient and his family to have an opportunity to visit the unit prior to admission, to meet staff and to have a glimpse of his fellow patients. Many adolescent units are in the grounds of mental hospitals and patients and parents may well have understandable anxieties about accepting admission. These may, or may not, be allayed by discussion, but at least the family's decision for or against admission may have some basis in reality after such a visit. In some units, this visit is combined with a measure of assessment regarding the patient's suitability for admission, but others prefer members of staff to visit the patient and his family at home before the introductory visit. Where the admission can be planned beforehand, either of these approaches may be satisfactory and in many units now there is an admission conference involving members of the multi-disciplinary staff team, a form of contract being worked out between the staff of the unit, the patient and his family. Occasionally, however, a planned admission may not be possible and the psychiatrist or another professional member of the team, has to make a decision about an immediate emergency admission, for example, where a teenager is considered to be actively suicidal, or acutely psychotic. Even here the reason for admission, whether it be need for help with a specific problem or a whole area of adolescent development, is usually discussed with the patient and family concerned.

The reasons for admission to hospital are various. The teenager may have become a danger to himself or to others; he and his family may be temporarily incompatible; or admission can be part of a prolonged treatment programme, as referred to above. For most youngsters, once the anxiety relating to admission is allayed there is a period of respite. They are content to find out how the unit functions and to acquaint themselves with staff and patients. The pressures of the outside world have abated temporarily and parental concern is likely to have taken on a positive quality, even where attitudes have previously been largely adverse. This is the period when the teenager is particularly receptive to new ideas and can re-examine his most pressing problems with staff help. He usually recognises quickly the standards of behaviour which are accepted and tolerated on the unit, but may then commence to test these out. It is essential that all staff should have an awareness of these processes and respond appropriately to them. At this stage also, the adolescent begins to form relationships which will be an important part of his treatment in the unit. These relationships are with staff and with his peer group.

STAFF

Whilst the psychiatrist, psychologist and social worker continue to have a role in the in-patient setting, the key members of the treatment team are the nurses, the teachers and the occupational therapist (if available). In the majority of hospitals, staff are appointed to work specifically on the adolescent unit and will naturally have indicated an interest in dealing with this age group. They will not be perfect; they will have normal human failings, but on the other hand, they will have a sensitivity to the teenager's needs, and an awareness of their own limitations and emotionally sensitive areas. Their satisfaction will lie in helping their patients to improve in all areas of achievement, rather than being confined to their own short-term goals. Staff members are used by teenagers as identification models and will have to come to terms with the roles which some of their patients will project upon them. They learn when to be firm and yet accepting, and it is important that the staff team provides a variety of personality and experience, so that children from many social backgrounds can be at ease. It is highly undesirable that units should project a middle-class, or indeed any specific class, image.

THE PATIENTS

Although a long waiting-list is undesirable, there may be some merit in having a short one, so that selection of the next admission can take into account the needs of the current group of in-patients. When a group consists of many acting-out, conduct-disordered teenagers, dilution with a more inhibited patient may be beneficial to all concerned. If the group has too many social isolates, the admission of a more extroverted teenager at this stage may be valuable. In a unit which covers a fairly wide age-range, it occasionally happens that there is a large group of younger patients and the older patients may not find each other's company congenial. In these circumstances treatment may be much more difficult.

TREATMENT PROGRAMME

A question commonly asked by parents of a prospective patient is, what kind of treatment will he be undergoing? Will he be having drugs or E.C.T.? Sometimes they are not convinced by the explanation that actually being in the unit is treatment, but nevertheless, this is the case. From the moment the patient is admitted until the time that he is discharged, the staff continuously observe and monitor his progress. In many units, these observations are fed into regular, often daily, staff meetings, attended by nurses, teachers and other staff-members, so that a detailed picture is built up about how the individual patient reacts in a group situation. Information so obtained is then used with the patient in a variety of ways to help him modify his behaviour. The child who antagonises his age-peers is helped to see the way in which this occurs and how he might modify his attitudes to become more acceptable. The patient who presents with marked feelings against authority should be given graded responsibility and be gradually helped to identify with authority, and to work along with its representatives. How these things are done varies from unit to unit. In some, use is made of large-group therapy as discussed previously, a privilege system may be employed or the patients themselves are encouraged to report on their observations of own or other patient's behaviour to the staff—patient group, so that the antecedents and repercussions of a particular episode can be analysed in a way which is helpful and supportive to the patient concerned. In other units, more use is made of individual psychotherapy. A combination of methods may be used. Whilst details of treatment vary from unit to unit and from time to time the overall emphasis of treatment is that it should occur within the total milieu and that that milieu should be beneficial.

Whilst the majority of teenagers can be treated in adolescent units, as has been mentioned, sometimes treatment on an adult ward may be preferable. This is particularly so for the very depressed teenager, particularly if he is regarded as actively suicidal and requiring constant supervision. In this instance, other teenage patients may be jealous of the staff attention which is being given and may label the suicidal patient as 'staff pet'. In such circumstances, the support given by adult patients may be more helpful. Not infrequently, the teenager has considerable difficulty in distinguishing between notoriety and fame and occasionally a teenager's behaviour may get out of control and is reinforced in an unhealthy way by the admiration he is receiving from his peer group. In order to help the patient regain a degree of self-control, adult support may be expedient. An acutely psychotic youngster may be frightening to other teenagers, who may have the understandable concern that they themselves may go 'out of their minds'. To alleviate their anxieties, they may ostracise the acutely-ill teenager, who can have sufficient insight to be aware of this rejection. Again, in such instances direct admission to an adult ward may be appropriate, transferring the patient back to the adolescent unit when his acute symptoms have come under control. Whilst the majority of mentally-subnormal teenagers requiring in-patient treatment are treated as special hospitals for the mentally subnormal, not infrequently a retarded patient is admitted for one reason or another to an adolescent unit and a decision will then have to be taken as to whether he should be protected from the gibes of the patients who are better endowed intellectually, or whether he will gain from their company. Sometimes, these patients are admitted to adult wards as a matter of policy, when the emotional pressure on them is likely to prove too severe.

In addition to the general approach to treatment just described, therapy specifically directed at the teenager's illness, as outlined in the preceding chapters, is also instituted when he is admitted to hospital.

With an increased awareness and improved training of the psychiatrist in the needs of adolescent patients, and with the increasing availability of out-patient treatment, the number of adolescents requiring in-patient treatment should remain small. As yet, no reliable studies on the prognosis of adolescent patients receiving out-patient treatment are available, but a number of studies report the prognosis of adolescents who have received in-patient treatment. Usually, it seems that in almost every diagnostic category, with the outstanding exception of the conduct-disorders, one-third make a good adjustment on their return to the community, one-third do more or less badly and one-third have only a precarious adjustment. Those patients with conduct-disorders being treated in hospital are obviously a highly selected group. It is difficult to evaluate the findings in this group at follow-up, but it certainly appears that they do significantly less well than those in other diagnostic categories. Methods and assessments are improving, but much remains to be done to improve the results of treatment of adolescent patients, particularly those who have marked conduct-disorders.

REFERENCES AND FURTHER READING

Easson, W. M. *The Severely Disturbed Adolescent*. The National Universities Press Inc., 1969.
Holmes, D. J. *The Adolescent in Psycho-Therapy*. Part III, page 245, seq. Little, Brown & Co. Boston, 1964.
Garber, B. *Follow-Up Study of Hospitalised Adolescents*. Butterworth, London, 1972.
Warren, W. 'A Study of Adolescent Psychiatric In-Patients and the Outcome Six or More Years Later.' Journal Child Psychol. and Psychiat., 1965, 6, pages 1–18 inclusive and 141–60 inclusive.

22 Conclusion

The majority of adolescents enjoy robust health, both physical and mental, and it is important to emphasise that only a minority experience serious psychological difficulties. The largest number within this minority presents to the local authority Social Services Departments and only a few reach the psychiatrist. On the whole, the referral seems to be relatively satisfactory, largely distinguishing between those who are sick and those who are simply in distress, although, in some instances, the division may only be paper-thin.

There are no psychiatric illnesses which are specific to adolescence, but the way in which some of the difficulties present may have a peculiar emphasis in response to teenage culture. The psychiatrist has to take into account the disturbed adolescent's developmental progress, in addition to his illness, in much the same way as the paediatrician has to assess the child's physical, mental and emotional development. He has to recognise that progress in treatment will be slow. He must be aware of the teenager's undue sensitivity at all times and has to help him to acquire a viable self-image. He needs to provide support and control, yet like the good parent, allow scope for experimentation and encourage initiative. Altogether this is a tall order which makes work with adolescents both challenging and frustrating, always trying to be a step ahead of the patient and yet knowing that one never will be. In a sense, the therapist suffers growing pains with each patient.

It is salutory to recollect that, over two thousand years ago, views concerning youth were much like those of today, even if couched in rather different terms. 'This youth is rotten from the very bottom of their hearts. The young people are malicious and lazy. They will never be as youth happened to be before; our today's youth will not be able to maintain our culture.' Little progress has been made in smoothing the path for adolescents and this task must be passed on to the present generation of teenagers, so that, as they become adult, they may, in their turn, aid the following generation of adolescents and take a more constructive view of youth than did the anonymous Babylonian writer quoted above.

Envoi

The average reader is anxious to get into the body of a new text and has little patience to read acknowledgments. Thus, although it is customary for these to be recorded at the beginning, it seems more appropriate that they should come at the end. I therefore record my thanks, as a tail-piece, to all those who have helped to bring this 'offspring' to maturity and would like to express my appreciation to Alistair Munro, formerly Professor of Psychiatry at Liverpool University and now Chief Psychiatrist at Toronto General Hospital, and to David Sutherland of Macdonald and Evans (Publishers), whose joint brain child this particular series is (*Psychiatric Topics for Community Workers*). The conception of this 'offspring' must be credited to Professor Munro, but both he and Mr. Sutherland have been equally responsible, as good parents, for the nurturing environment provided for its development and have at all times coped with the author's 'growing pains', so that support and reassurance were always readily forthcoming and yet there was no undue repression.

My gratitude is also expressed to the several typists who have helped with the production of the manuscript, tolerating the illegible scrawl and the unintelligible noise from the dictaphone, to family, friends and colleagues who accepted a degree of disruption of their plans uncomplainingly, and to Elizabeth Jamie, Elizabeth O'Brien and David Turland for helpful comments and encouragement.

Finally the author is indebted to those who have contributed to her professional nurture over the years and on whose original thinking and research she has drawn so heavily in this text.

Index

305

Lourie, R. 90
Low birth weight 4
Lukianowicz, N. 206

Maladjusted
definition 44
schools for the 144
see also Schools
Marks, I. 160, 263
Marriage 154, 155, 191, 196, 210, 219
in schizophrenia 69
Mason, P. 135
Masterson, J. 51, 77
McCord, J. 134
McCord, W. 134
McCulloch, J. W. 48
McWhinney, A. 228
Medical model xii, 40, 239
Medical officer, clinical (formerly school) 36, 85
Medlicott, P. 175
Memory 39, 60, 159, 169, 170, 262
Mendel, G. 7
Meningitis 55, 56, 215
Menstruation 22, 23, 24, 160, 180, 190
Mental handicap 7, 41, 49, 221–6, 279, 287–8, 300
Mental Health Act 1959 73, 89, 107, 143
Mental illness
general 135
parental 14, 41, 46–7
Mental state 39, 55
Mental subnormality
see Mental handicap
Mental Welfare Officer 37
Meyer, V. 273
Mitchell, S. 50
Mixed conduct and neurotic disorder 128
Mongolism (Down's Syndrome), 6, 224
Moniz, E. 262
Monk, M. A. 160
Mood disturbance
anxiety 51, 159, 180
see also Anxiety
classification of 72
depression 50, 51, 72, 74–82
elation 50, 63, 72–4, 50–82
general 39
Moral values 31
Morris, D. P. 152
Mother
see Parents
Mother, unmarried 198, 229
Multi-disciplinary staff team xi, 297
Myoclonic seizures 212
see also Epilepsy

Nail biting 171
Narcosis 171
Nervous system and neurological disorder 5, 134, 157, 215
Neurotic disorder 40, 41, 43, 50, 138, 157–71
Newson, E. 9, 10
Newson, J. 9, 10
Non-attendance at school 43, 174–84
see also School
Nursing care 292

Obsessional-compulsive neurosis 43, 115, 164–9, 263
Obsessional symptoms 43, 76, 115, 164, 181, 228
Offences 130
sexual 206
Olsen, T. 77
Oppenheim, A. W. 50
Organic disorder 40, 135, 167, 223
Orientation 39, 54, 56
Ounstead, C. 125, 228

Paediatric ward 15
Paediatrician 152
Paedophilia 206, 277
Parents
absence 13
anxiety in 90, 171
attitudes of 12, 17–18, 140, 180, 188
background 13, 132, 133
death of 13–14, 78
disharmony 14, 47, 154, 155
divorce 14, 136
general 13
illness 13, 47, 70
lone 13, 14, 47
relationship to child 11–18, 180
separation of 14
Parkinsonian side-effects 250–1
Pasamanick, B. 5, 123, 134
Pavlov, I. P. 273
Peel, E. A. 25
Peer-group relationships, 30, 180, 183
Perceptual disturbance 54
Personality
affective 153
anancastic (obsessive-compulsive) 154
anti-social (psychopathic) 155
asthenic (inadequate) 155
change in 57, 61
classification of 152
definition of 3
dependent 150
development 115, 147–52
disorder 40, 41, 43, 50, 115, 138, 152–5
explosive 154
hysterical 154
in depression 78
in schizophrenia 69
paranoid 153
schizoid 153
Petit mal seizures 213
see Epilepsy
Phenylketonuria 7
Phobias 165–6
social 109, 161, 274
Physical development
in childhood 111, 152
in adolescence 20–3
see Adolescence, physical development
Physical differences between the sexes 20–4
Physical handicap 209–21
Physical illness 135, 174–5, 179
Piaget, J. 25, 140, 151
Police 36, 44, 130, 143, 207
Poverty
see Environment, material